Who is Molly

Who is Molly?

Molly Drug Facts, What is Ecstasy, and Life-Saving MDMA Effects Info

by Taite Adams

Who is Molly

Rapid   Response   Press
6860 Gulfport Blvd., Suite 357

St.   Petersburg,   FL   33707
www.rapidresponsepress.com

Ordering   Information:
Quantity sales. Special discounts are available on quantity purchases by corporations, associations, and others. For details, contact the publisher   at   the   address   above. Orders by U.S. trade bookstores and wholesalers. Please contact Rapid Response Press: Tel: (866) 983-3025; Fax: (855) 877-4736 or visit www. rapidresponsepress.com.

Printed in the United States of America

Publisher's   Cataloging-in-Publication   data
Adams,   Taite.
A title of a book : a subtitle of the same book / Taite Adams.
p.   cm.
ISBN :9780988987593   978-0-9889875-9-3
1. The main category of the book —Health —Other category. 2. Another subject category —Mind and Body. 3. More categories — Recovery.

First Edition

==================

Taite Adams

Limit of Liability/Disclaimer of Warranty

Limit of Liability/Disclaimer of Warranty: While the publisher and author have used their best efforts in preparing this book, they make no representations or warranties with respect to the accuracy or completeness of the contents of this book and specifically disclaim any implied warranties or merchantability or fitness for a particular purpose. No warranty may be created or extended by sales representatives or written sales materials. The advice and strategies contained herein may not be suitable for your situation. You should consult with a professional where appropriate. The publisher and author do not assume and hereby disclaim any liability to any party for any loss, damage, or disruption caused by errors or omissions, whether such errors or omissions result from negligence, accident, or any other cause.

For general information on our other products and services or for technical support please contact Rapid Response Press - 6860 Gulfport Blvd., Suite 357; St. Petersburg, FL 33707

================

Disclaimer

Disclaimer: This publication is designed to provide accurate and personal experience information in regard to the subject matter covered. It is sold with the understanding that the author, contributors, publisher are not engaged in rendering counseling or other professional services. If counseling advice or other expert assistance is required, the services of a competent professional person should be sought out.

==================

Medical Disclaimer

The information contained in this book is not intended to serve as a replacement for professional medical advice. Any use of the information in this book is at the reader's discretion. The author and publisher specifically disclaim any and all liability arising directly or indirectly from the use or application of any information contained in this book. A health care professional should be consulted regarding your specific situation.

To my Son - Thank you for keeping the conversation going;

To Mom - Who kept telling me over and over and over again not to do drugs - I finally get it;

To my Love - The more time that I have with you the more I don't ever ever want it to end - what a blessing we have been given.

Get All The Books In The Series:

Kickstart Your Recovery - The Road Less Traveled to Freedom From Addiction

Safely Detox From Alcohol and Drugs at Home

Opiate Addiction - The Painkiller Addiction Epidemic, Heroin Addiction and The Way Out

Restart Your Recovery

For More Information, visit http://www.taiteadams.com

Table of Contents

Preface

Most people that hear about "Molly" on the news or through the grapevine think that we are being assaulted by a "new" drug. I know I did. Being the mother of a teenager and someone who has had a dialogue going with their child about drugs for years, I have been hearing about Molly for quite awhile now. What surprised me was twofold. One - is that the drug itself really is nothing new, just brilliant re-branding and marketing on someone's part. Two - was the massive amount of misinformation that is being passed around about the drug, not just from teen to teen and then on to concerned parents, but also through trusted media outlets. A lot of the information being disseminated is just flat out wrong, irresponsible and frankly dangerous. As someone who has been in recovery from addiction for many years, I have had my fair share of experience with drugs, including "club drugs". While Molly made be a reincarnate of the club drugs of old in some form, there is also something much more insidious and dangerous about it that the public needs to be made aware of. While the purists of the bunch insist that Molly is a safe high and free from adulterants, nothing could be further from the truth.

Who is Molly

Drugs are a bet with your mind. - Jim Morrison

Molly is all over the news, the internet and even being pushed by some of today's biggest celebrities. Parents, teachers, policymakers and the curious are looking for more information about this "new drug". There is so much information about Molly being passed around, little doubt that a lot of it is misinformation and hastily gathered facts and figures. What is lacking is a single source for Molly drug and MDMA information that separates fact from fiction. This book about Molly aims to do just that - Learn about Molly and MDMA Facts, Ecstasy History, Molly Effects, Dangers of Molly Use and Overdose, Molly Addiction and Detox, and Talking to Your Teen or Loved One About Molly in the following pages.

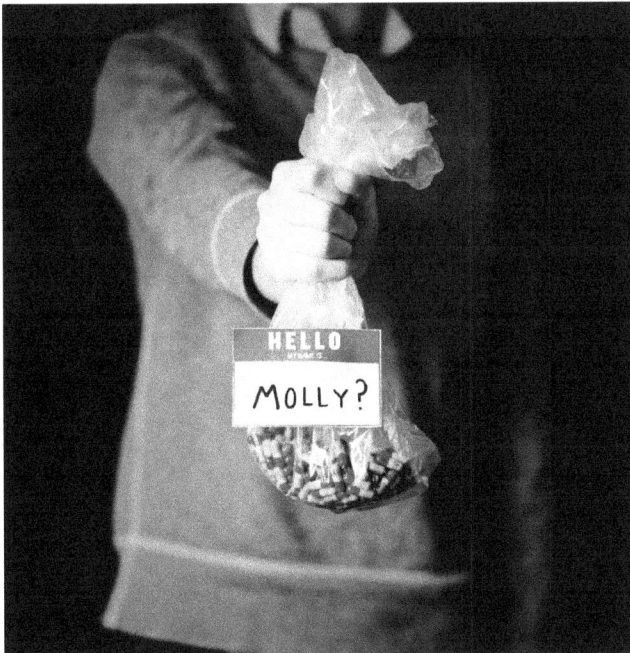

Molly Drug Facts

Pain could be killed. Sadness could not, but the drugs did shut its mouth for a time. — Colson Whitehead

Let's get the number one misconception out of the way first. Molly is NOT a "new" drug - not by a long shot. Molly is simply the re-branded form of Ecstasy (though not the same as Ecstasy) for the new generation. Short for "molecule", it is the powder or crystalline form of MDMA, or 3,4-methylenedioxy-N-methylamphetamine. Typically sold in either a pressed pill or capsule that is taken orally, or as a crystalline powder that is snorted or swallowed, a Molly dose generally lasts from 4-6 hours. Sometimes the pressed pills can have cartoon-like images on them and some people take more than one pill at a time, called "bumping". Molly is considered somewhat cheap, with a street price of around $20-$40 for 100mg, which is typically enough for a first time user.

Molly, or MDMA, is an entirely synthetic drug and is part of the amphetamine family. It is classified as a Schedule I substance, meaning that it has no recognized medicinal use and is considered to have a high abuse potential. The DEA has said that the purity of Molly is almost a myth because it comes in powder form and can easily be mixed with other drugs, making it infinitely more dangerous. DEA officials have also stated that the drug is mainly manufactured in Canada, Asia and the Netherlands and is much more complex to make than meth.

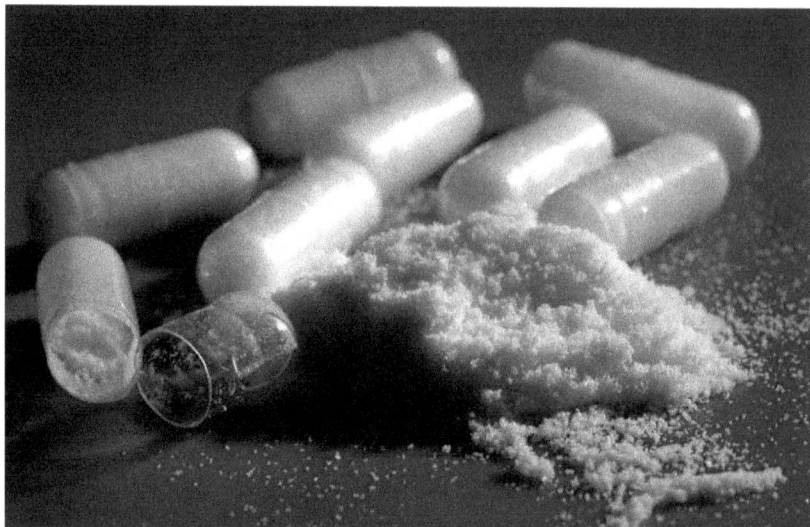

A 2010 U.N. World Drug report estimated that around 10-25 million people used Molly at least once per year. A comparison of the 2012 and 2013 Global Drug Surveys, conducted by an independent drug-use data agency, shows just how popular Molly has become. In 2012, 26.5 percent of U.S. respondents had tried MDMA in the last 12 months. In 2013, the number jumped to 60.9 percent. Typical settings for Molly use are dance clubs and music festivals where there is a high level of stimulus, as the drug enhances visual, sound, smell and touch stimulation. These heightened sensations make people on the drug want to dance, touch and talk even more.

The biggest misconception with Molly, and this will be discussed in more detail later, is that it is "purer" than other drugs, even its ancestor "ecstasy". This couldn't be further than the truth as many powders and pills being sold as Molly contain little to no MDMA in them at all, being simply mixture of various harmful synthetic contaminants thrown together to meet the skyrocketing demand for this popular drug. "Anybody who propagates the idea that this is purer than anything else— it's ridiculous," says Dr. Julie Holland, a psychiatrist in private practice and the editor of Ecstasy: The Complete Guide, "It's a white powder. What could be more of a question mark? At least in a tablet someone put some time into putting it together. But [the name Molly] sounds so innocent, like a girl in freckles and pigtails. It's good marketing."

No, Molly isn't really "new" at all. But the perception that it is and that it's the "purest" form of MDMA makes the drugs prospect scary. When we talk about Ecstasy and other "club drugs", most know that there are many risks involved. The key is to disseminate this same sort of information about Molly. Ecstasy has a long enough history of use and abuse that a clearer message can be formed about this drug.

What is Ecstasy and It's Long History

History never looks like history when you are living through it. -
John W. Gardner

We say that Molly is just Ecstasy re-invented for the new generation, but this is only partially true. In fact, Molly is simply the newest and, to date, the most pure form of MDMA. In theory, anyway. MDMA itself was first "invented" in Germany in 1912 by the Merck Company, and then patented in 1913. They never did much with it, briefly considering its use as a diet pill and then scrapping all plans. There are rumors of the drug being "tested" by the U.S. Army in the 1950's as a possible truth serum, but not much evidence to support this.

Dr. Alexander Shulgin, of U.C. Berkeley and later Dow Chemical, is considered to be the man responsible for the modern research of MDMA in the 1970's. A biochemist, Shulgin is considered the first "reported" human to use the drug and report his findings in detail. During the 1970's, in the United States, some scientists began using MDMA as a psychotherapeutic tool, despite the fact that the drug had never undergone any FDA trials for use in humans. Despite this, the drug gained a small fan-based amongst psychiatrists in the late 1970's and early 1980's, with some calling it "penicillin for the soul" because it was considered to enhance patient communication during sessions and allowed patients to achieve insights that had previously alluded them.

Who is Molly

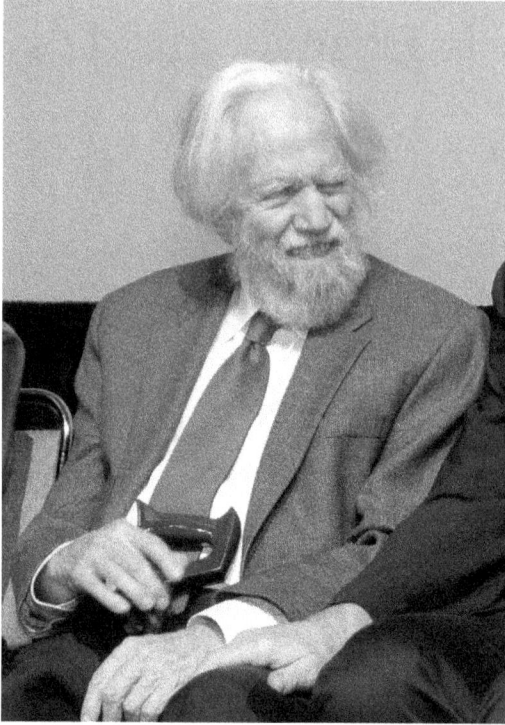

By 1977, both a powder and pill form of MDMA had quietly emerged as a recreational drug in both the U.S. and the U.K. In 1982, the Hacienda, a former warehouse turned nightclub, opened its doors in Manchester, England and this pioneered the "Madchester" scene and a pioneering Ibiza party, hosted by DJ's Mike Pickering and Jon DaSilva known as "Hot." The club's following grew feverishly and with it, a reputation for hard party drugs. In the 2002 film "24 Hour Party People", real-life Mr. Manchester Tony Wilson (played by Steve Coogan) comments: "This is it. The birth of rave culture. The beatification of the beat. The dance age. This is the moment when even the white man starts dancing. Welcome to Madchester."

Then, in 1984, former seminary student and self-proclaimed "Ecstasy missionary," Michael Clegg returned to Dallas from a religious experience in California with a group of therapists. He brought MDMA with him, hooked up with some chemists, and started his own manufacturing operation. He sold it at clubs and through a 1-800 number (even offering free-shipping). One particularly popular club, just off the Woodall Rodgers Freeway, was the Starck Club, frequented by celebrities like Grace Jones and Stevie Nicks. "You had sexual freedom, which had come out of the '70s, and the drug culture was still going on," says filmmaker Michael Cain. Cain is currently in post-production for a new documentary, The Starck Project, about the club — which is regarded by many as the birthplace of rave culture in America. "It was just what you did...almost like a pyramid scheme. People would get invited to parties and be asked, 'Would you like to buy it? Would you like to sell it to your friends?' You could make money   doing   this."

Before long, rave culture emerged throughout the world, fueled by DJs, LSD, and a psychoactive that became known on the streets by many names: Molly, Ecstasy, Adam, Disco Biscuits, Malcolm X, Scooby Snacks, and Skittles. "Nobody called the drug MDMA. Everyone said 'x-tasy' or 'X,'" says Michael T, a DJ, promoter, and fixture at popular Manhattan club The Limelight throughout the '80s. Up until that point, MDMA bore many nicknames, but it was all the same   substance   —   and   it   was   loved.

Then, in 1985, the government began a crackdown on MDMA, and it officially became a Schedule I controlled substance. Good, bad or ugly, this is where things really took a turn and MDMA became "Ecstasy" as we know it today and much more dangerous than ever before.   As supply dwindled, demand surged, and thus, an underground economic incentive was created to form cheaper manufacturing methods. Ecstasy took on a new meaning. A new pressed-pill form of MDMA was born. It was cut with other, cheaper substances, like caffeine, cocaine, ketamine, or fertilizer.

By the early '90s, with rave culture in full trance, popular scare tactics emerged from many drug researchers insinuating that Ecstasy would put permanent holes in the user's brain, or even connecting it to early-onset Parkinson's (this controversial statement was retracted soon after). In 2000, Time magazine jumped on the bandwagon, scaring the bejesus out of parents around the country with its cover story "What Ecstasy Does To Your Brain." In it, 18-year-old "Karen" revealed that "the cliques are pretty big in [her] school, and every clique does it." And thus the warning bell was sounded.

In 2002, the RAVE Act ("Reducing Americans' Vulnerability to Ecstasy") increased penalties and mandatory minimum sentences. But that hasn't stopped the scene from going and growing strong, nor the re-birth of a "purer" form of the drug for the next generation. Until, again, demand surges and adulterants move in.

Dangerous Molly Propaganda

"How many people in this crowd have seen Molly?" - Madonna

The recent deaths and overdoses we hear about on the news aren't the only things that are contributing to the rise of Molly's popularity. Depending on your taste in music, references to the drug are rampant. Here are just a few examples:

"We like to party dancing with molly/Doing whatever we want"   Miley Cyrus - "We Can't Stop"

"Something about Mary, she gone off that Molly/ Now the whole party is melted like Dalí"   Kanye West - "Mercy"

"Hi, I'm looking for Molly I've been searching everywhere And I can't seem to find Molly, Molly, Molly, Molly, Molly, Molly, Molly, Molly Molly, Molly, Molly, Molly, Molly, Molly, Molly, Molly (Fucked around and fell in love with her)" Tyga ft. Wiz Khalifa & Mally Mal - "Molly"

"Palms rise to the universe/ As we moonshine and molly/ Feel the warmth, we'll never die/ We're like diamonds in the sky"   Rihanna - "Diamonds"

"We pop a molly, she buss it open"   French Montana - "Pop That"

"I'm in molly world, I need a molly girl Pineapple swirl, keep me in molly world Right now because I'm bussin', feel on top of the world I'm out here off a molly, I need a molly girl I'm in molly world, I'm in molly world Bitch I'm out here bussin', I need a molly girl I'm in molly world, I'm in molly world Bitch I'm off the shits, I need a molly girl"   Lil Durk ft. Wiz Khalifa - "Molly Girl"

Who is Molly

"Please help me find Molly./ Hi I am looking for Molly/ I've been searching everywhere and I can't seem to find Molly/ Do you know where I can find Molly/ She makes my life happier/More exciting/ She makes me want to dance" Cedric Gervais - "Molly"

"Just popped a molly with Miley/She do shrooms every blue moon" Childish Gambino ft. Schoolboy Q & Ab-Soul - "Unnecessary"

"Got your girl on molly and we smokin' loud and drinkin'/ Got my top back so you can see what I been thinkin'" Nicki Minaj ft. 2 Chainz - "Beez In The Trap"

"She popped a Molly I'm guessing But if she throwing the pussy I'm catching" Trinidad James ft. 2 Chainz, T.I., Young Jeezy - "All Gold Everything Remix"

"I see molly is the new cocaine" Wyclef - "Hip Hop"

"Where that bitch that do that molly and that bitch to roll my weed/ Don't get no molly in my blunt but put this molly on your tongue/Watch your eyes get wide and your tongue get numb/Oh sweat dance turn up" Problem ft. Gunplay & Trinidad James - "My Last Molly Song Ever I Promise"

"Pop a molly now that bitch sweatin'" Rick Ross - "Box Chevy"

"Iceberg vest, I'm sniffing molly of a chess board" Sir Michael Rocks ft. GLC - "You Know The Rules"

"Let's take it back to the first party/ When you tried your first molly/ And came out of your body" Kanye West - "Blood On The Leaves"

"She got that feeling, feeling/ Shorty be twerking off the pill/ Her clothes start peeling peeling/ This ain't no joke these girls for real/ She touched the ceiling ceiling/ She bought that party here for real/ I call her molly molly/ She brought that party here for real" French Montana ft. Meek Mill & Wiz Khalifa - "Molly"

"Put molly up in her champagne, she didn't even know it / Took her home and I enjoyed that, she didn't even know it" Rocko ft. Future, Rick Ross - "U.O.E.N.O"

"Sell your momma a zip of dust/Serve your daddy a ounce of hard/ Got your little sister on the molly/ She done went through the whole squad" Gucci Mane - "Trap Back"

"Fucked around and popped a Molly, now I'm high as fuck" Snoop Dogg & Wiz Khalifa ft. Juicy J - "Smokin On"

"She wanna pop a molly man, Juicy J gon' fuckin let her" Wiz Khalifa ft. Juicy J - "T.A.P."

"Fuck the world with my thumb/Pop a molly, smoke a blunt/That mean I'm a high roller" Nicki Minaj ft. Lil Wayne - "Roman Reloaded"

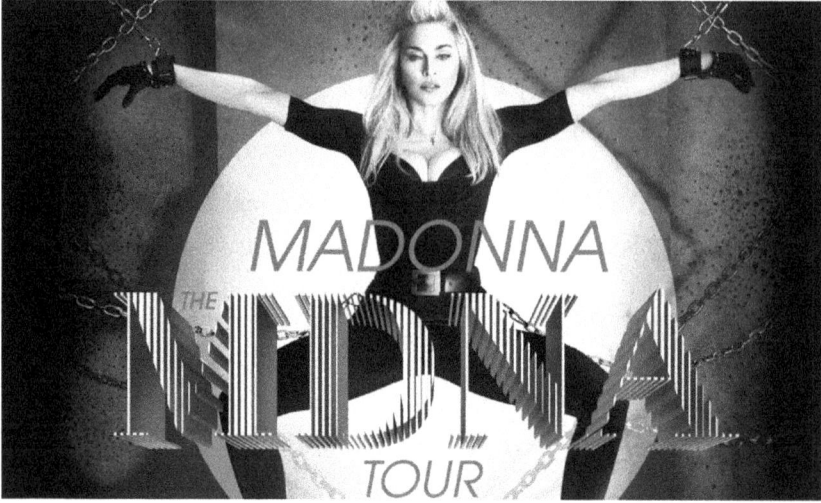

This isn't all of them and the hits will keep "rolling" out as long as we keep buying. Is there really anything we can do about the celebrity propaganda of drug use? Well, maybe not but there are a few stories that aren't being told in these songs that probably should be.

Why Celebs Are Saying Molly is Cool

Selling my soul would be a lot easier if I could just find it. — *Nikki Sixx*

Celebrity references to drug use aren't new by any means and this new cycle of MDMA, coined "Molly", is just the latest. However, it has been getting a great deal of attention in the media and several celebrities have seen some serious backlash as a result of their propagandizing drug use. Madonna not only questioned her Miami, FL Ultra Music Festival audience about "seeing Molly", she also named her latest album "MDNA". After getting flak over this, she backpedaled with some ridiculous excuses that don't even make sense.

Cedric Gervais has stated that his song is actually "about a girl named Molly that makes him want to dance". Ok. Miley Cyrus, who was once a powerful role model to young girls, is another story. Her publicist has stated that her song lyrics are actually "dancing with Miley", while Miley herself says, "no, it's Molly". We see and hear Lil Wayne rapping about Molly in many songs but most don't know that he's been arrested multiple times on drug charges and is now drug tested regularly. No Molly for him. Rapper Rick Ross learned a valuable lesson when he lost a multi-million dollar Reebok endorsement after rapping about putting Molly in a girl's champagne.

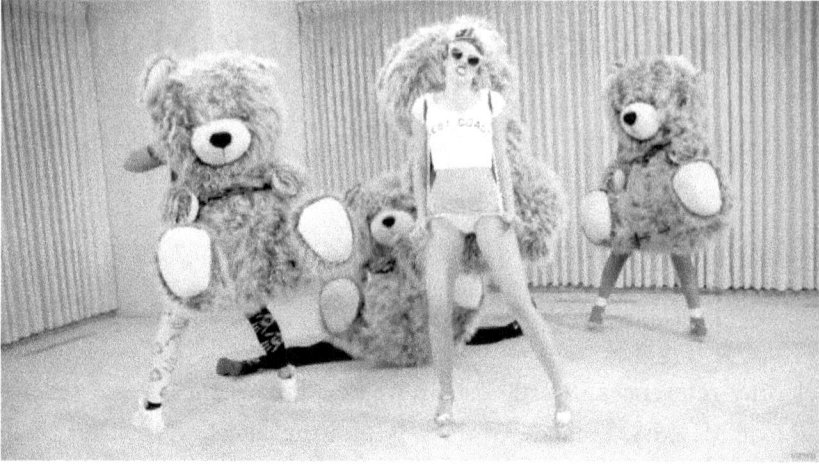

Celebrities, especially hip hop artists, are going to continue to say that Molly is "cool" until the next big thing comes along. The fact that more mainstream artists, like Madonna and Cyrus, are touting the drug is troubling as it creates a potentially toxic combination for younger, female music fans. Christopher Crosby, CEO of Florida-based addiction treatment facility, The Watershed, agrees. "Young fans are more likely to try drugs if they see their idols doing it, but it's more than just the use of drugs – it's the emotion behind the use," he said. "If these teens are in a place where they are looking for acceptance and a sense of belonging, they will most likely be at a greater risk of drug abuse."

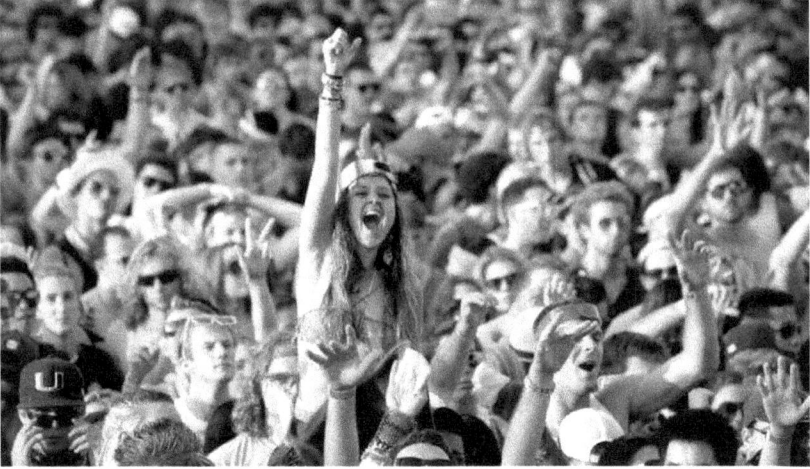

In fact, celebrity references to Molly use could be building a comfort zone for many who were reluctant to try the drug before, turning what they considered to be something potentially dangerous into something "safe" or ok. Young adults might think it's alright when seeing celebrities such as Madonna referring to the drug especially at such a large event. As the drug's popularity increases, more college students, young adults, and even teenagers feel that it's ok to experiment when they attend music festivals and parties. Many are still not aware of the potential effects of the drug or versed on safety considerations.

I've never had a problem with drugs. I've had problems with the police.   *-Keith   Richards*

Molly and MDMA Effects Explained

Real knowledge is to know the extent of one's ignorance. - Confucius

Trying to outline the effects of Molly, the effects of Ecstasy and MDMA effects is tricky business because they are not one and the same. People who think that they are getting Molly, oftentimes are not and this has become one of the biggest dangers of the drug. Ecstasy has long been known to be a virtual hodge podge of chemicals and fillers, with MDMA being only a staple ingredient. However, one errant dose of ketamine or fertilizer can be a real buzz kill. Hence the dilemma. So, let's take a look at all of these factors as systematically as possible. First, looking at the effects of just MDMA, then long-term effects of Molly and Ecstasy use. Finally, a few words on safety considerations that could be the difference between life and death.

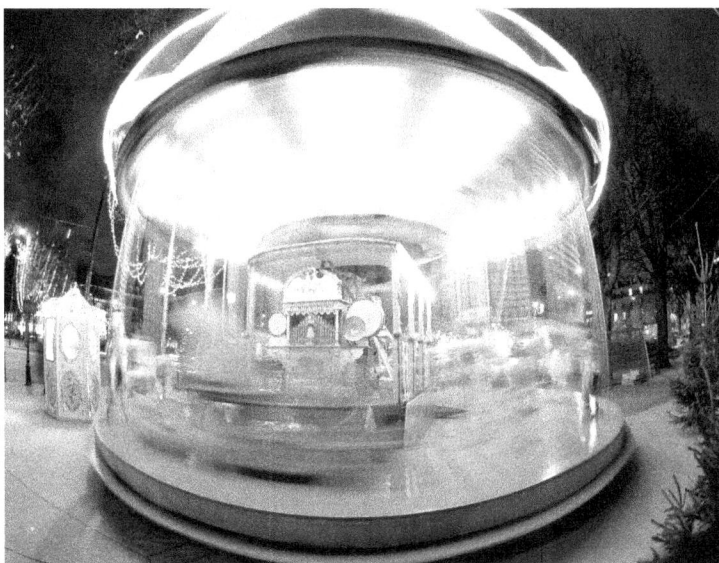

The Effects of Pure MDMA

Beware of false knowledge; it is more dangerous than ignorance. -
George Bernard Shaw

MDMA (3,4-methylenedioxy-methamphetamine), is a synthetic,
psychoactive drug that has similarities to both the stimulant
amphetamine and the hallucinogen mescaline. MDMA produces
immediate feelings of increased energy, warmth, euphoria, and feelings
of closeness and empathy as a result of a surge in serotonin,
norepinephrine, and dopamine. Users typically experience an altered
sense of perception, as well as time and space. Side effects can include
dehydration, anorexia, feelings of anxiety as well as "bruxism" or teeth
grinding.

The drug's massive release of serotonin can have other consequences,
such as the potential to result in a deadly condition known as serotonin
syndrome, characterized by hyperthermia, rigid muscles, along with an
altered mental status or confusion. Serotonin also triggers the release of
the hormones oxytocin and vasopressin, which play important roles in
love, trust, sexual arousal, and other social experiences. This may
account for the characteristic feelings of emotional closeness and
empathy produced by the drug; studies in both rats and humans have
shown that MDMA raises the levels of these hormones. The drug's
release of the hormone called ADH (antiduretic hormone) or
vasopressin from the pituitary gland can also have negative effects, as
this hormone also controls water re-absorption and, if disturbed, can
result in hyponatremia (low serum sodium concentration) accompanied
by swelling of the brain and resultant seizures.

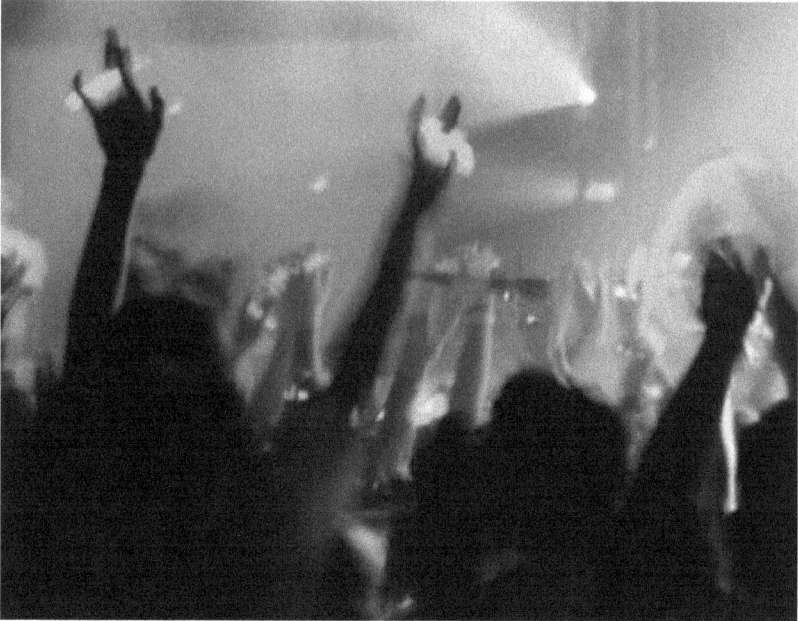

MDMA, even in its pure form, can produce elevated heart rates and distortion of thought processes, causing users not to realize their rising body temperature or fading stamina as they continue to party. The drug has a dangerous side effect profile which can be lethal due to sharp elevations of blood pressure, coupled with cardiac arrhythmias, intractable seizures, as well as extreme elevations in body temperature (hyperthermia).

Theodore Bania, a medical toxicologist and emergency medicine physician at St. Luke's-Roosevelt Hospital in New York, said although many of the people who take Molly don't end up in the emergency room, some users experience side effects that land them in the hospital. Bania frequently sees patients who have complications from MDMA, ranging from dehydration and exhaustion to more severe side effects such as hyperthermia, seizures, electrolyte abnormalities, cardiac episodes and comas.

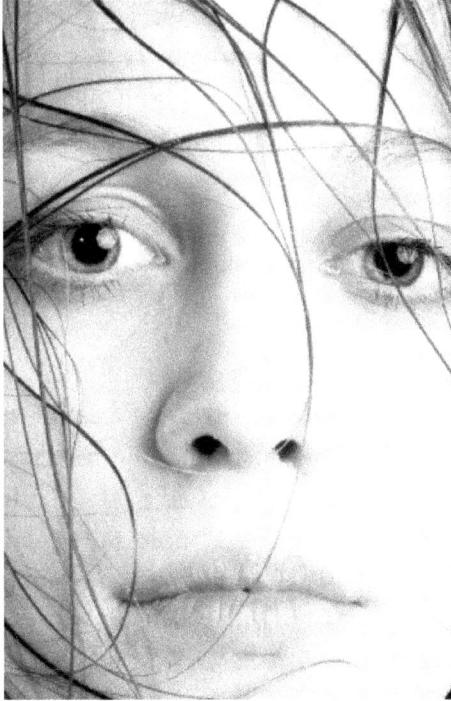

MDMA also depletes the body of some of its neurotransmitters, which can lead to a decreased mood about a day or two after using the drug. Some experts have stated that they have even seen use of the drug lead to long-term depression. Before we even discuss long-term, the laws of physics state that what goes up must come down and "Suicide Tuesday" is the term coined for the massive bout of depression that can follow 1-2 days after using MDMA due to the massive drop in serotonin. This needs to replenish on its own and can take anywhere from 48 hours to a week.

Who is Molly

The first time Adam tried Molly, he was 19. He loved it. "I was visiting friends in Boulder for a Sound Tribe Sector 9 show at Red Rocks," says Adam, who was raised in Chicago. Twenty minutes before the concert started, he was popping a nondescript pill. At first, he felt nothing. But as the concert continued, the colors of the stage became amplified and his feelings of self-consciousness slipped away. "I was happy. I started to just smile and dance to my own drum," he remembers.

Adam's comedown experience, and that of many other users, was horrific. He became "tweaky" in his movements - grinding his teeth uncontrollably and licking his lips. When he tried to go to sleep later that night, he couldn't. "It was impossible. My mind was racing and I was super aware of my surroundings - noises my friend was making on the couch, lights flickering. I felt paranoid," he recounts.

Users who haven't had exposure to molly's serious negative side effects sometimes think of it as a "safer" drug. But Carl Hart, an associate professor of psychology at Columbia University, said claims that any drug is safe are ridiculous. "A lot has to do with the doses people take," Hart said. "As you increase the dose over an extended period of time, you can expect to see some negative effects. That's a general rule the public really needs to understand."

Hart said he believes accurate education, not law enforcement, is key to minimizing the risks of illicit drugs such as Molly. Because so many young people have already tried Molly, he said experts need to make sure they are being realistic about the dangers of its use, including potential long-term effects.

Molly and Ecstasy Long Term Effects

Never take ecstasy, beer, baccardi, weed, pepto bismol, vivarin, tums, tagamet hb, xanax, and valium in the same day. It makes it difficult to sleep at night. -Eminem

Many people love to tout the "safety" of Molly and it's purity but that has become pure nonsense. Although we'll get into this more when discussing safety and overdose considerations, the fact of the matter is that when you "use Molly", you will be more than likely also ingesting a host of other chemicals into your body and, if you do this on a repeated basis, there will be long-term effects. Ecstasy is differentiated from Molly because it is "cut" with other adulterants. Well, that is exactly what Molly has now become due to the unscrupulous dealers trying to meet a massive spike in demand. So, what happens when you roll with this stuff long-term? Some long-term effects of MDMA are debatable, others are pretty much a given.

Long-term use of MDMA can result in what is called "MDMA Neurotoxicity". Large and frequent doses of MDMA can destroy serotonin axons. Serotonin neurons (brain cells) form a sort of control system in your brain, regulating emotions, appetite, sleep and other functions. The serotonin axons are 'communication cables' that the serotonin system uses to send its signals to the rest of the brain. (MDMA works primarily by causing these serotonin axons to release a lot of serotonin at once, causing euphoria.) Animal experiments suggest that if neurotoxicity occurs, some new serotonin axons can grow to replace them... but they grow in different places than where the original ones were.

The long-term effects of this 'rewiring' are not known. Although there is considerable debate over how much MDMA it would take to cause damage to a human user's brain, there is no real doubt that at some dosages damage can and will occur. This neurotoxicity, changes in the brain, discussed above, could manifest itself in a range of symptoms such as: depression, sleep and memory problems., anxiety, emotional instability, and trouble concentrating.

There were some scare tactic media stories about a decade ago claiming that MDMA causes Parkinson's Disease by damaging the dopamine system. The story and underlying study were later retracted as being completely false. There have also been allegations about MDMA causing "holes in your brain". This isn't entirely true. What is does cause is a reduction in blood flow in the brain for a period of time, which is what shows up on a brain scan and makes it appear to have "holes". Is a reduction in blood flow to your brain an acceptable effect from using a drug? Still - No!

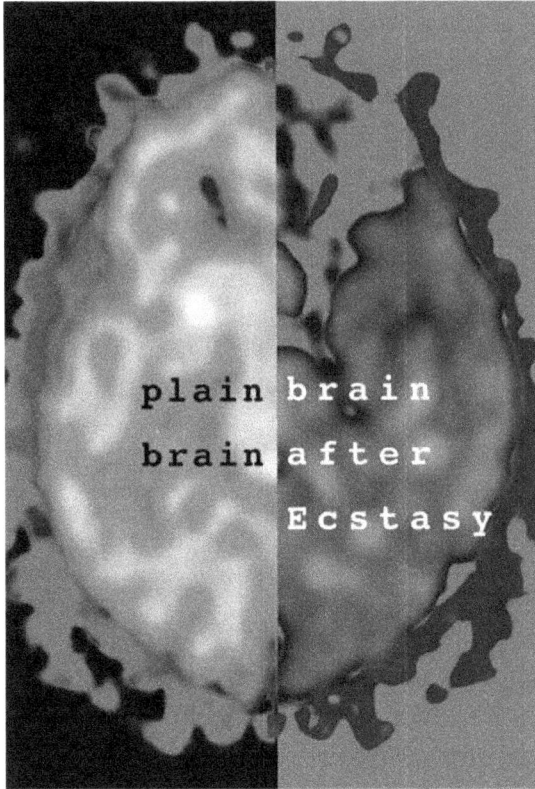

plain brain
brain after
Ecstasy

Another factor to consider with regards to the long-term effects of Molly and Ecstasy are other serotonin issues and depression. While some may bounce back from the "Tuesday Blues" fairly quickly, others find themselves simply stuck in a lingering depression after using MDMA. The release of serotonin, also causes serotonin receptors in the brain to down-regulate, which basically means turn themselves off for a while. The up-and-down regulation of receptors is one of the primary ways the brain tries to achieve homeostasis, or balance. These receptors work in conjunction with the amount of serotonin around and are just as important in the regulation of mood as serotonin itself.

In trying to maintain a balanced mood, these receptors respond to the amount of serotonin around by turning themselves on and off (up-regulation and down-regulation). When they are flooded with serotonin as a result of taking Ecstasy, many of them down-regulate.

The majority of these receptors will up-regulate again as soon as the excess serotonin is metabolized away. However, some of these receptors may stay down-regulated longer, perhaps days, weeks, or even months. The depression some people feel after taking ecstasy may be a result of these serotonin receptors staying down-regulated too long.

Finally, some users of MDMA and ecstasy may have simply been depressed before ever picking up the drug. Some even find that the feeling experienced with the drug allow them to self-medicate their depression which, in the end, may exacerbate the symptoms of the depression and cause many more problems in the long term.

This wouldn't be complete without mentioning that, when using any of these drugs in high doses and long term, you are not just exposing yourself to the long-term effects of MDMA but to whatever adulterant the dealer felt was worthy of tossing in the pot that day, whether it be meth, cocaine or some other research chemical.

Molly Safety - Both Sides of the Debate

There is no safety in numbers, or in anything else. -James Thurber

Is Molly "safe"? Ten years ago, it might have been a moderately safe bet if you were forced to pick an illicit drug to put to into your system and marijuana was taken off the table. Not anymore. It's popularity has literally killed it's safety and there is no longer a difference between Molly and Ecstasy. In theory? maybe. In reality - not at all and those of us reading and buying books of this sort are attempting to stay planted firmly in reality.

The drug that is "pure MDMA" is now fallacy and, as soon as people wake up and realize this and the dangerous that it represents, demand will fall. "The No. 1 risk with MDMA is drug substitution," says Julie Holland, a New York University psychiatry professor who has run trials investigating MDMA's therapeutic potential. In legitimate markets, increasing demand tends to improve quality; with illicit drugs, it does exactly the opposite. "For the longest time, we would almost never see something sold as Molly that wasn't," DanceSafe's Board President Nathan Messer says. "It was like a cottage industry comprised of relatively ethical psychedelics manufacturers. They liked MDMA, and they wanted other people to be able to have it." But now that Molly is such a hot commodity, its strongest selling points - purity and a worry-free roll - are exactly what are being exploited by dealers.

As Molly's popularity skyrockets, the ability to regulate it becomes nearly impossible: a fact that officials say results in "bad batches" of

Molly which can contain anything from meth to heroin to cocaine. In a massive bust last August in the college town of Syracuse, New York, the $500,000 worth of Molly that police seized contained no MDMA at all. The incident prompted a group of students to launch a website debunking Molly as an urban legend. Regardless, many will continue to buy it and use it and there are important safety considerations for those that insist on taking this route.

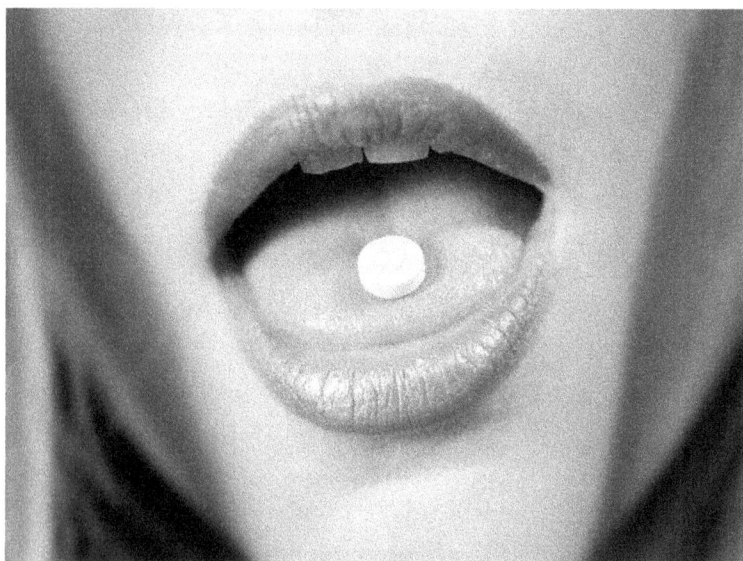

Increased risks develop when users mix the drug with alcohol, synthetic cannabinoids, (K2 or Spice) or especially cocaine which contributes to its increased potential for toxicity. This means that after you take Molly, you shouldn't be ingesting these things on top of it. As far as what is actually in that Molly pill that you're about to pop, there's really no way to be 100% sure. You can buy a test kit (see Resources Section) that will allow you to test whether it has any MDMA in it at all, but it's not always going to tell you if it's cut with meth, research chemicals or fertilizer. These kits are still highly recommended.

Take care of yourself by staying hydrated at the proper level. Overhydration is very dangerous and can lead to death. Stick to 8-16oz of water or sports drinks per hour. Don't redose, or "bump", as everyone's body chemistry is different. Don't be afraid to ask for help if you feel you are in a dangerous place. You won't get in trouble. Get valuable information about Molly overdose warning signs in the next chapter.

Molly and MDMA Overdose Facts

It ain't what you don't know that gets you into trouble. It's what you know for sure that just ain't so. -Mark Twain

The most significant problem faced with users of Molly, MDMA or Ecstasy - and really one of main points I'm trying to get across with this book - is the uncontrolled quality of the pills. Most of the time, the pills contain something along with the MDMA (such as research chemicals, meth, cocaine, etc). Still others contains no MDMA whatsoever and are sold as "Molly".   They may contain other research chemicals such as MDPV, methylone or mephedrone or simply have a mix of drugs in them, like meth.   In one awful case back in 2000, a group produced a batch of a drug called "PMA" and sold it as MDMA, causing an estimated twenty deaths worldwide.   As you can imagine, the dangers for overdose and death with this drug are very real. Skeptical? Recent events speak for themselves.

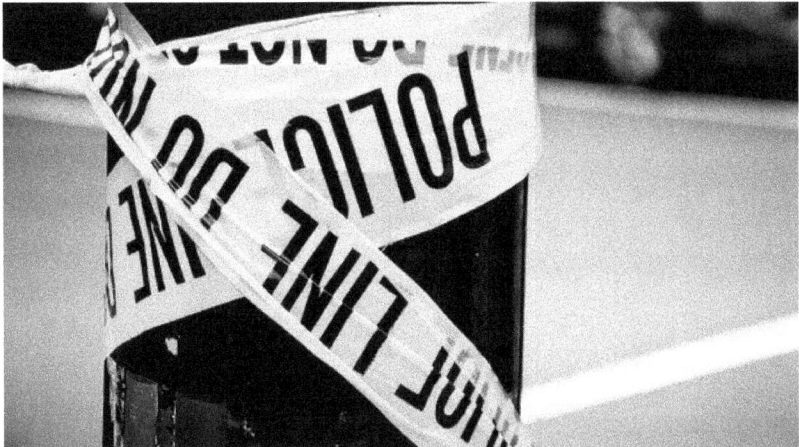

Molly Overdose Incidents and Deaths are Climbing

If we don't change our direction, we are likely to end up where we are headed. -Ancient Chinese Proverb

If ever in doubt about the growing popularity and "danger" of a particular illicit drug, frequency of stories about it in the media can generally shed some light. Molly has been receiving its share of attention for several years now but the rise in media stories about its use, its propaganda and its dangers have skyrocketed in 2013. And for good reason. As [music] festival season settled onto the Summer of 2013, there was a marked change in atmosphere from recent years. Molly and ecstasy have always been present to an extent, but nothing like the numbers we are seeing now. The resulting dangerous substances flooding the market have brought a new level of crisis to communities and heartache to families.

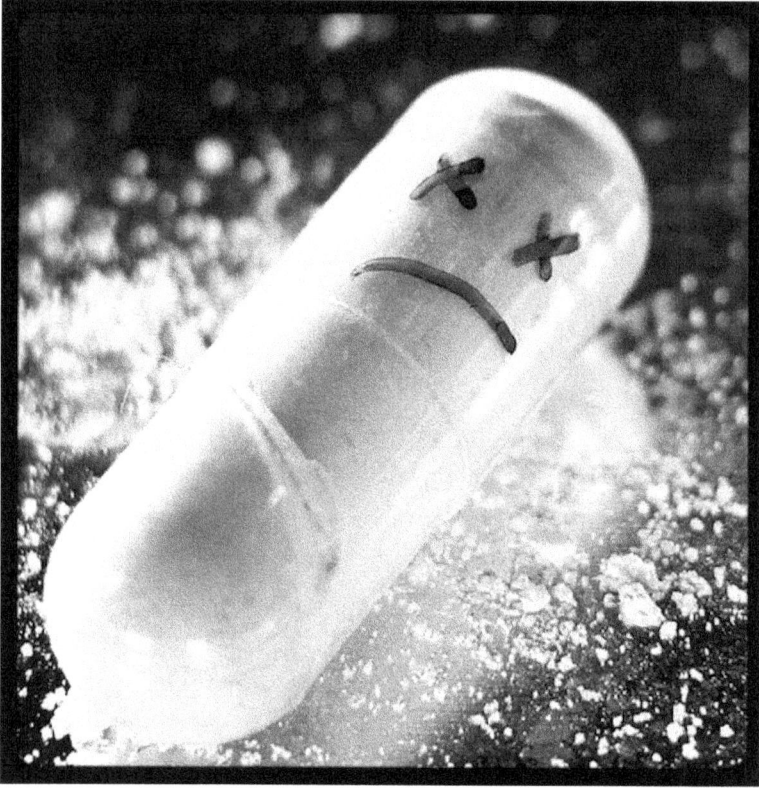

Police suspect that a poisonous batch of Molly may be responsible for the death of a teenage girl at Boston's House of Blues on August 27th, the deaths of two Electric Zoo attendees who died over the weekend, and many other non-fatal Molly overdoses across the Northeast. At the Electric Zoo festival in New York City, University of New Hampshire student Olivia Rotondo collapsed into a seizure on Saturday and later died after allegedly taking six hits of Molly. Syracuse University graduate Jeffrey Russ, 23, also died as a result of drug use following the concert.

19-year-old Brittany Flanigan's final hours at Boston's House of Blues were described by the Boston Globe: *One woman had fallen down on the dance floor, but told security she was fine. She wanted to go back to the concert, and refused medical treatment. But when she tried to walk away, her body suddenly went stiff. A short time later, 19-year-old Brittany Flannigan, was found "convulsing on her feet," a security employee said. Her older sister by her side, Flannigan was taken to a stairwell, where she lay down. But the convulsions wouldn't stop. "We just tried to stay with her until the ambulance came," said William Farago, a security staffer who had been at the scene.*

Flannigan was later pronounced dead, with tainted Molly believed to be the cause. Two other people at the club were also treated for suspected overdoses, and days later another two Boston concertgoers survived suspected Molly overdoses at a Sound Tribe Sector 9 concert. This summer more than a dozen ambulances were called to respond to Molly overdoses at the Ocean Club in Boston's Marina Bay.

At least six people in Scotland died over the summer from a tainted batch of Ecstasy, and in July, a message board user claiming to be a worker in a Vancouver toxicology lab warned of a fatal batch of Molly in the area, and theorized that PMMA mixed with MDMA was responsible:

"In case you're not familiar with PMMA: it's a molecule closely related to MDMA, but with much less of the desired empathogenic/euphoric effect, and unfortunately quite a bit more toxicity. The dose curve is a lot steeper, and the effects are delayed compared to MDMA. Often what has happened in these fatalities is that somebody takes one or two pills, and doesn't get the expected effect, so takes more, and that's enough to push them over into the toxic range. The toxicity looks basically the same as an overdose of MDMA, causing serotonin syndrome. Symptoms might include: Fast heart beat, overheating, excessive sweating, shivering, headache, involuntary twitching of the legs, twitching of the eyeballs... It's important to mention that the recent deaths have been caused by PMMA mixed with

MDMA, not PMMA alone. This means that pill testing kits (from Dancesafe, etc.) can't pick them up! They will show a normal purple/black reaction because of the MDMA mixed in."

This past summer in Seattle, one man died and many more were treated after overdosing on Molly at the Paradiso music festival at the Gorge Amphitheatre in central Washington, authorities said. Patrick D. Witkowski, 21, of the Seattle suburb of Des Moines, died Sunday at Central Washington Hospital in Wenatchee. An autopsy found no physical injuries or pre-existing medical conditions that would have caused the death, Harris said. Sarina Fahrner, the chief nursing officer at Quincy Valley Medical Center, told reporters that there were more than 100 overdose patients from the same music festival.

In September 2013, A University of Virginia sophomore died after collapsing at a District nightclub over the holiday weekend. 19 year-old Mary "Shelley" Goldsmith, an honors student from Abingdon, VA was at a rave concert at a club called Echo Stage in D.C. Robert G. Goldsmith said his daughter's friends told him that she had taken Molly. He said family members discussed whether to make the information public and concluded that they had to warn others. "Shelley deserves a legacy of being someone who cared for people, someone who achieved, someone who contributed, and not a druggie who died," he said. "That's not who she was. But if her death can open someone's eyes, then we need to talk about it."

There are warning signs of overdose and contributing factors that anyone who is in close contact with this drug should be familiar with.

Factors Contributing to Overdose

It is during our darkest moments that we must focus to see the light.
-Aristotle Onassis

The number one factor contributing to overdose is the fact that you probably have no clue what you just put in your body. Many users will find that they aren't getting the desired "MDMA effects" from whatever they've taken and just take a bunch more. This can have disastrous consequences. Nathan Messer, board president of the nonprofit organization DanceSafe, which promotes health and safety within the nightclub community said MDPV, methylone, mephedrone and butylone -- different substances or drugs -- are often sold as Molly. In fact, here is a list of just a few of the substances that could be in that pill:

MDA: This cousin of MDMA is very similar in affects, but has been described as 'more psychedelic'. Test kits can determine if a pill contains MDA instead of MDMA. (Pills containing a mixture of MDMA and MDA are somewhat common.)

MDEA: MDEA is another cousin of MDMA. Test kits cannot distinguish between MDMA and MDEA.

Methamphetamine: METH is a powerful and relatively dangerous stimulant drug. The home test kits can identify pills that contain METH by itself, but not METH combined with one of the other MDxx drugs. According to the US Drug Enforcement Agency, about 2.5% of 'ecstasy' pills contain a mixture of MDMA and METH, while 3% contain only METH.

DXM (dextromethorphan): This legal cough syrup ingredient is also seen with some frequency. It's psychoactive at high doses. A test kit can usually identify a pill containing DXM.

Ketamine: Rarely sold as 'ecstasy', Ketamine is a sedative used for veterinary surgery. It used to be used for humans as well, but FDA approval was withdrawn after patients began reporting having hallucinations while they regained consciousness. Test kits do not identify ketamine.

Caffeine, Ephedrine, Psuedoephedrine: Seen with some frequency, these ingredients are relatively inactive unless taken at very high doses.

Legal Psychoactives: Occasionally legal (research) chemicals like 5-MeO-DIPT and piperazines have been sold as 'ecstasy', but this is likely to end with the recent banning of these drugs in the US.

PMA: para-MethoxyAmphetamine is rarely seen, although there was a small seizure of gelcaps containing PMA in the US in early 2004. The last time a large batch of PMA hit the streets, it killed about 20 people. The main problem seemed to be that it took over an hour to kick in (vs. 30-40 minutes for MDMA), so users would think they had gotten weak pills when nothing happened in the first hour, take a few more, and overdose.

Heroin: Some dealers claim such a thing is common - it's really not.

LSD, cocaine, mescaline: LSD and Mescaline have never been found in 'ecstasy' pills. There have been a few isolated cases of pills containing cocaine and MDMA (and a few pills containing only cocaine that might be mistaken for 'ecstasy' tablets.) Cocaine actually counteracts MDMA (it blocks the serotonin transporters) so it simply doesn't make sense to use it as a cut; meth is cheaper and more effective.

Natalie, a 23-year-old interior designer, now understands this all too well. Her first experience with MDMA - or what she thought was Molly - ended with her in the fetal position for 48 hours, shaking and vomiting intermittently between hallucinations of evil faces flying at her. It wasn't until days later, when Natalie recovered, that she heard the news. A girl who'd rolled from the same batch she did ended up in the hospital. Toxicology reports revealed that the drug (which had the "consistency of powdered sugar") wasn't Molly at all - it was meth.

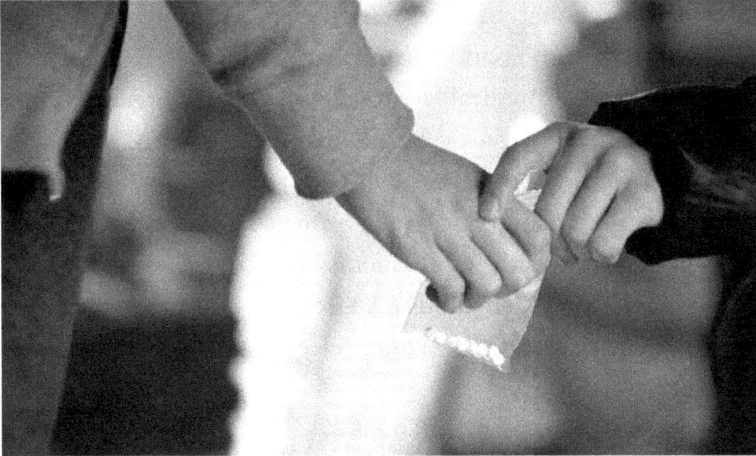

The data collection site, ecstasydata.org calculated that only 23 percent of the samples of Molly sent in by consumers and tested in its DEA-licensed lab in 2013 were actually pure MDMA. In response to the recent wave of bunk drugs, a group called "The Bunk Police" began selling test kits online, and setting up tables at events, so people could test what they are buying to see if it is actually safe. The most common adulterants in the samples tested by "The Bunk Police" this summer were the synthetic drugs known as bath salts, including the cathinones

MDPV, methylone and mephedrone. The following message can be found on their website:

Nearly 100% of substances are cut with one or more adulterant, and they aren't using baking soda anymore. Over half of samples tested by our group contain large quantities of "research chemicals" of multiple classes and types, many of which present very real overdose risks and have been in news reports all over the world.

Despite these very real risks, there are still overdose risks from MDMA and its combination with other substances. The Drug Abuse Warning Network's study also found that from 2004 to 2009, there was a 123% increase in the number of emergency room visits involving MDMA taken alone or in combination with pharmaceuticals, alcohol or both. Theodore Bania, a medical toxicologist and emergency medicine physician at St. Luke's-Roosevelt Hospital in New York, said although many of the people who take molly don't end up in the emergency room, some users experience side effects that land them in the hospital. Bania frequently sees patients who have complications from MDMA, ranging from dehydration and exhaustion to more severe side effects such as hyperthermia, seizures, electrolyte abnormalities, cardiac episodes and comas.

Signs and symptoms of ecstasy and MDMA overdose include:

- Headache
- Blurred vision
- Chest pain
- Dry mouth
- Nausea, vomiting
- Abdominal cramping
- Urinary retention
- Sexual dysfunction
- High blood pressure
- Panic attacks
- Feeling faint

- Loss of consciousness
- Increased body temperature
- Seizures
- Stiffening of muscles
- Insomnia
- Depression
- Paranoia

While ecstasy is unlikely to cause death due to overdose, it can cause very unpleasant symptoms. Muscle cramps are common, as are problems urinating or sweating. The most serious symptom of an MDMA overdose is overheating - when the body enters a state of hyperthermia, various organs and tissues can be damaged very easily. The inability to sweat is a precursor to this. Overweight people may be more susceptible to hyperthermia, and MDMA can be particularly dangerous for anyone who has existing medical conditions like asthma or other respiratory issues.

With continued use of the drug – especially in crowded and hot settings – the potential for dehydration increases, forcing users to continuously consume large quantities of water, further compounding the risks of developing hyponatremia, as a result of water intoxication. Hyponatremia means "low salt" and results from drinking too much water, too fast. Deaths have occurred from this and it is a very real danger at even low doses of MDMA and just moderately high fluid intake.

Ecstasy can be particularly dangerous when taken with other drugs, because MDMA can inhibit a drug user's ability to limit him or herself. A person on MDMA may take much larger amounts of other recreational drugs than what that person would normally take, leading to other forms of overdose that are complicated by the MDMA still in the drug user's system.

Some medications and other recreational drugs don't mix well with MDMA. Here's a brief list of drugs and concerns:

Drug:	Issues:
Amphetamines (speed, crystal meth, etc.)	Mixing MDMA with other amphetamines increases the risk of heatstroke, hypertension, heart attack and death. Mixing amphetamines may also increase the risk of neurotoxicity, which is highly dependent on overheating to occur.
Alcohol (and other sedatives such as GHB, etc.)	Can greatly increase the degree of intoxication while making the user less aware of it. Large amounts of alcohol mixed with MDMA can produce bizarre behavior with no memory of it the next day. Mixing stimulants and depressants can allow the user to unwittingly take dangerously large amounts of either since they counteract each other's effects. There have been some unexplained deaths involving mixing alcohol and MDMA. Most people that end up in the emergency room after using MDMA were mixing it with alcohol.
Cannabis (marijuana) and hashish:	If used simultaneously the two drugs may not mix well and/or interfere with each other. Smoking a large amount of pot while high on MDMA can be counterproductive and unpleasant.
LSD	The combination of LSD and MDMA is popularly called "candyflipping." Beware: These drugs are synergistic (a small amount of MDMA and a small amount of LSD can have a strong effect when taken together.)
Psilocybin ("Magic Mushrooms")	Called "Hippieflipping", effects might be amplified by mixing with MDMA (like LSD.)
Cocaine	Cocaine aggressively competes with MDMA for access to the neurotransmitter transport proteins. There have been a fair number of deaths involving MDMA and cocaine mixing

Who is Molly

Drug:	Issues:
Prozac, Zoloft, Paxil, other SSRIs and SNRIs	Drugs that inhibit serotonin reuptake (often prescribed for depression, anxiety, trouble sleeping, etc.) will block MDMA's ability to work. The degree of interference varies by person, SSRI, and dose, but as much as a 70% loss of MDMA's effects seems to be common.
Adderall	See Amphetamine.
Viagra (sildenafil)	Viagra is sometimes taken by ecstasy users to overcome the common problem of impotence in men while under the influence of MDMA. Viagra actually causes a drop in blood pressure, not an increase. Viagra is not completely safe even by itself; around sixty deaths were reported in the first year of its availability.
MAOI drugs	**Never** combine MDMA with an MAOI. **M**onoamine **O**xidase **I**nhibitors prevent the breakdown of neurotransmitters like dopamine and/or serotonin (depending on the type of MAOI.) As a result, dopamine/serotonin levels can become dangerously high if an MAOI is combined with drugs that release dopamine/serotonin (such as MDMA.) MAOIs have sometimes been prescribed for depression; if in doubt, ask your pharmacist if a medication you are taking is an MAOI.
DXM (Dextromethorphan.)	Commonly found in cold and cough medications, DXM is sometimes used recreationally (it is hallucinogenic at high doses.) DXM may reduce your body's awareness of overheating, and interferes with the breakdown of MDMA by competing for the CYP2D6 enzyme.
Caffeine, Ephedra, Psuedoephedrine.	Stimulants used for alertness, weight loss and as decongestants, these drugs increase pulse and blood pressure. Combining them with other stimulants may increase the risk of heart attack, stroke, heatstroke.

If you notice the symptoms of an ecstasy overdose, you should contact a physician as quickly as possible, especially if you believe that the chances of hyperthermia are high in the drug user. If an overdose situation does occur with Molly, what someone assumes to be Molly, or its combination with other substances, you may not get in trouble but do expect to be questioned so that you can be helped.

When an emergency medical response team deals with an MDMA overdose, they will often ask for as much information about the patient's drug use as is possible. Therefore, collecting information about what the overdosed drug user took can be very helpful. However, this can be easier said than done, as overdoses can cause people to become confused or unconscious. Nevertheless, any attempt to gather information about drug use will be helpful, and if you're able to give the medical response team a sample of the drug that was used, it may improve the chances of successful treatment. Medical personnel may discuss several topics with you or your loved one before treating ecstasy and MDMA overdose symptoms. These topics include:

- Patient's age, weight and physical condition
- Time the drug was taken
- How much of the drug was ingested
- Other substances that were ingested

Medical personnel will initially want to stabilize your respiratory function and open your airway if necessary. Assistive devices may be used to do this. Because ecstasy and MDMA overdose symptoms commonly include paranoia, doctors may take precautions to ensure you don't try to escape medical care. Intravenous fluids are often administered to prevent dehydration caused by hyperthermia. Other treatment methods may include:

- Gastric lavage
- Activated charcoal
- Administration of medications to treat hypertension and agitation
- Cool baths to treat hyperthermia

There are no agonists or other medications that can be given as antidotes to ecstasy and MDMA. Supportive care is continued until your ecstasy and MDMA overdose symptoms have ceased. Most patients recover fully within seven hours.

After an MDMA overdose occurs, drug counseling or addiction counseling may be necessary. Drug addiction treatment can help to prevent another overdose from occurring, and you should consider this if you or someone you know has recently overdosed on ecstasy.

Is Molly Addictive?

The priority of any addict is to anesthetize the pain of living to ease the passage of day with some purchased relief. — *Russell Brand*

Like many other drugs, MDMA (or Molly), can absolutely be addictive. That is, people continue to use the drug despite experiencing unpleasant physical side effects and other social, behavioral, and health consequences. While some people may be more susceptible than others, no one knows how many times a person can use a drug before becoming addicted to it. As with other drugs of abuse, a person's genes, living environment, and other factors play a role in whether they are likely to become addicted to MDMA.

Molly is a scheduled I substance because it is not only illegal but has a high potential of abuse. While many people do not develop chemical dependency on Molly, psychological craving with MDMA (the defining characteristic of addiction) can be quite high. Because Molly is a recreational drug, addiction is more likely when you take MDMA for effect. However, addiction and physical dependence are two separate clinical conditions. Dependence happens when the body has adapted to the continued presence of MDMA in the system and presents withdrawal symptoms once you stop taking it. Prolonged abuse of Molly can completely alter the brain chemistry to the point that cognitive behavior is only normal with the presence of the drug inside the body. At this point, the body is physically addicted to Molly.

On the other hand, addiction may be present because the added psychological element of seeking out Molly even though it is hurting your body or your life may be more likely. Addiction can also involve seeking out the drug to self-medicate and mitigate the lack of pleasure and stimuli in your life. Simply taking Molly over time can lead to an addiction and negative relationship with the drug. Remember, Molly use is not regulated and so many do not know the level of doses it takes to become addicted. Nor is there any sort of tapering process that compensates for withdrawal or help the brain reach homeostasis. Therefore, it is hard to determine how fast someone can become addicted to Molly, especially with the many adulterants that are likely present in what you are taking. There are simply too many factors that play into it.

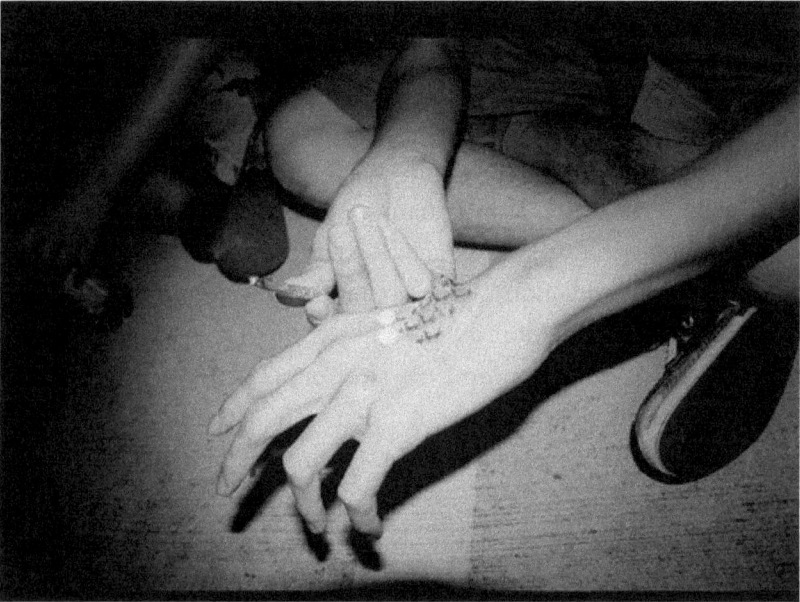

James, who lives in Pawtucket, RI, is currently in rehab for drug addiction. He said his choice of drug was Molly. "I was looking for ecstasy and they tell me we have a new form of ecstasy. You know it's just MDMA. It's more powerful. Why don't you try this? That's how I started," he said.

But James warns after the high, you crash hard. "Afterward you feel real dirty. You feel real dirty, tired and worn out. Coming off of it, it's no joke also. You have sweats especially when you're doing it. The dehydration is insane," he said. And do things you normally wouldn't do. "My wake up moment was when I found myself selling my little boys' video games to support the habit," James said.

Natalie Holmes from Atlanta wants to warn other young people about the dangers of Molly. She binged on the substance and was in and out of rehab six times in four years. "It's pretty prevalent and has gotten even worse since the last time I used it," she told local reporters.

The New Jersey rapper Joe Budden says he spent last summer binging on Molly and barely made it out alive. "I didn't see a problem with the fact that maybe five days would go by without sleeping," Budden told a Fox affiliate in New Jersey. "I didn't see a problem with the fact that maybe I was hallucinating at times. I didn't see a problem with the fact that I just couldn't get up and walk sometimes."

"It just altered your thinking process dramatically and for a thinker like myself that was like nothing I'd ever experienced before," says the MC, who's third studio album, No Love Lost, was released in early 2013. He says he kicked the habit with the help of his loved ones, and thinks it's important to speak up about his experience. "Now everyone is speaking about Molly like it's the thing to do," he says. "I thought it was important for somebody, anybody, to stand up and say, 'you know, I did that, it's corny.' I'm just hoping that at the end of the day, it won't be me versus the entire music industry when it comes to who a 13-year-old should listen to regarding drugs."

Who is Molly

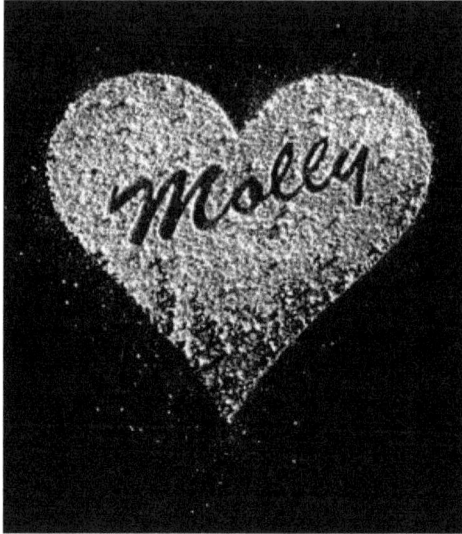

It's important to note that, everyone is different and reacts to Molly in different ways. Overall, continued abuse and self-medication using MDMA regularly will lead to addiction. Also, if you or your family have a tendency toward dependency to drugs or alcohol, you may be at a higher risk compared to someone who isn't. If you feel you may be addicted to Molly, look out for the signs and then seek professional help to support your decision to stay away from MDMA.

Again, chemical dependence to MDMA and Molly addiction can be similar but are clinically different conditions. However, if you think you may addicted to Molly, the following are good indicators of Molly addiction:

1. Using Molly in order to maintain normal function regardless of withdrawal
2. Seeking out Molly and disrupting your life to take it
3. Craving the drug
4. Rationalized use of Molly in order to continue taking it

If you or a loved one is experimenting with ecstasy in the night club or rave scene, yet cannot get enough of the drug; an addiction may exist. Drug addiction to "party drugs" can sometimes be difficult to recognize at first, but is a serious problem. The difficulty of detecting an addiction in "party drugs" is because one takes the MDMA in a social setting with many others approving their decision of ingesting the drug. If you do have a problem with Molly and MDMA, there are treatment facilities around the world that can assist you in overcoming your addiction and learning how to lead a drug free life.

Why do I act like I'm all high and mighty when inside I'm dying. I've finally realized that I need help. -Eminem

Ecstasy Detox Information

Your present circumstances don't determine where you can go; they merely determine where you start. -Nido Qubein

If you have become dependent on ecstasy, or MDMA, and wish to break free, the good news is that ecstasy detox itself is not life threatening. You will most certainly experience some unpleasant symptoms but, provided you are able to meet a few simple criteria and can make some simple preparations, you should not have any problem managing this at home. Also, ecstasy is not something that you "taper" or wean yourself off of. There is no benefit to doing this and it may cause more harm. You simply need to stop taking it and deal with the withdrawal symptoms until they pass. So, detoxing from MDMA at home is feasible provided you can meet these simple criteria:

- Have a safe, comfortable place to go through withdrawal symptoms, away from temptation.
- Not have a history of severe withdrawal symptoms or of trying and failing to withdraw at home.
- You have no co-occurring medical or psychiatric conditions that would require close observation during this period.

The onset of ecstasy withdrawal symptoms is going to vary wildly depending on your level of use - ie - how much you took and how often. For example, if you were taking MDMA around the clock, expect symptoms to start within 4-6 hours of missing your first dose. Symptoms that you are likely to experience include:

- Anxiety
- Insomnia
- Depression
- Irritability
- Memory problems
- Mood fluctuations

Also, because Molly now found in clubs is rarely 100% pure, you may have a concurrent addiction to some type of amphetamine-like substance that was mixed in (or "cut") with your MDMA. In this case, you will also experience some amphetamine withdrawal symptoms and may also need to do your research to get a better idea on how to manage them. Likewise, if you are abusing other drugs on top of MDMA, such as alcohol or cocaine, this complicates matters. If withdrawal symptoms seem severe and are too much to take (have another person there to be the judge), be sure to seek medical attention immediately. There is no shame in checking yourself in for a medically-assisted detox. Generally, symptoms are much more mild by day 5 or before and detox from ecstasy has not been found to be life threatening.

What is important to realize with Ecstasy withdrawal is that some level or form of symptoms can be felt for a very long time after you stop taking the drug - sometimes months or even years. Also, in the case of MDMA a lot of damage could have been done both physically and psychologically, sometimes permanent. Increases in heart rate and blood pressure are a special risk for people with circulatory or heart disease. "The serotonin system, which is compromised by MDMA, is fundamental to the brain's integration of information and emotion," says Dr. Alan I. Leshner, director of the National Institute on Drug Abuse (NIDA). "At the very least, people who take MDMA, even just a few times, are risking long-term, perhaps permanent, problems with learning and memory." While many issues can be repaired over time, it's important to stop use and soon as possible and deal with ecstasy detox in the safest and most responsible manner.

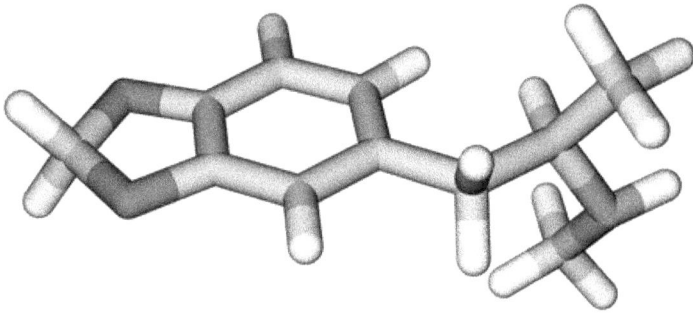

It is important that you make proper preparations for a detox from ecstasy by having the right support and supplies on hand. If you haven't lined up someone to stay with you, do this now. You really need someone staying with you from Day 1 with MDMA as the symptoms could start right away, are emotionally taxing and can last for quite a few days. Don't expect to go to work or probably anyplace while this is going on so have some things on hand to keep you occupied during the times that you are unable to sleep.

If you haven't set up an appointment with your physician to discuss your plans, also do this now. A long-acting Benzo (like Valium) can be a big help in detoxing from ecstasy. This is something that you will be on for a week, at the most, and on a reducing dose to deal with anxiety and ease some of the other withdrawal symptoms. If you are unable to get a prescription, that's ok. You can still find some comfort with over-the-counter medicines, supplements, vitamins and diet.

Here are some over-the-counter medications that you'll want to pick up and their uses:

- **Benadryl (Diphenhydramine)** - This one is recommended. This can help with anxiety, restlessness, and insomnia. Take 25-50 mgs every 6 hours as needed.
- **OTC Pain Reliever** such as Tylenol, Aleve, Aspirin or Ibuprofen for headaches.

As for vitamins and supplements, here are the things that you'll want to consider picking up if your budget allows (you had money for your drugs, didn't you?). Simply stick with the recommended dosages for all of these:

- Vitamin B
- Vitamin C
- Vitamin E
- Calcium
- Magnesium
- Thiamin
- Niacin
- L-Glutamine
- Milk Thistle (helps with liver repair)
- Valerian Root (very helpful for insomnia)
- Passion Flower

**If you can find the 1st five of these in a good multi-vitamin, that's fine too.

Aside from these things, how you treat your body from this point forward also has a lot to do with how the rest of your detox is going to go for you. While there may be periods of time where you have no or little appetite, diet is critical and having the right foods and beverages on hand is very important. You'll want to pick up lots of fruits and vegetables, whether they are your favorites or not. This is about replacing the toxins that are leaving your body with good things that are going to make you feel better, and Ice Cream or Doritos aren't going to cut it. With ecstasy detox, generally your appetite will increase. This is great because chances are you've been starving yourself and are massively undernourished right now. However, make the right choice and put some good things in your body for once. On the flip side, if you're not feeling well, it's ok to eat in small amounts but when you do eat something, eat the right things. Either way, stock up on some of this stuff:

- Fiber-rich fruits and vegetables
- Healthy proteins from chicken, fish and eggs
- Plant proteins such as beans and peas
- Healthy fats from fish
- Nuts, seeds, extra virgin olive oil

The intake of fluids cannot be stressed enough. It's crucial that you drink moderate to large amounts of water. Do not consume more than 2 quarts in an hour, however. It is ok to mix in a few sports drinks for flavor but try to stick primarily to water for fluid intake. You may also with to add some cranberry juice to the mix as it helps to purify and cleanse the body. Staying hydrated will help the withdrawal symptoms be less severe and allow the toxins to flush out of your system more quickly. Stay away from caffeinated drinks like coffee and tea. Your sleep patterns will already be very disturbed. These drinks will only exacerbate that and will not help to keep you hydrated.

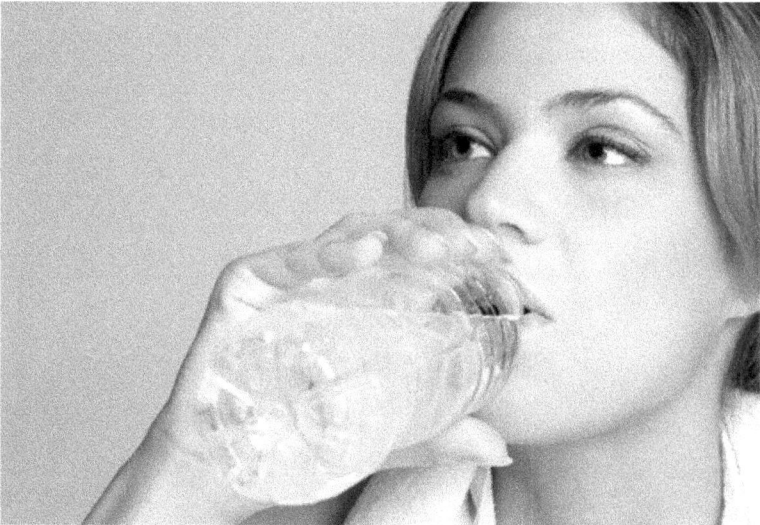

Finally, other things you'll want to do during ecstasy withdrawal to ease symptoms include taking frequent baths as this can help the emotions as well as the body. The water temperature should really be to your comfort - whatever is going to make you feel better and more comfortable at that moment. It could be the complete opposite just a little while later. Mild exercise, such as stretching and going for a short walk, may also help with circulation and anxiety through the release of endorphins. Releasing these natural "feel good" neurotransmitters can help to ease feelings of depression and anxiety. Rest when you are able and keep your mind busy when you aren't. When you can't sleep, keep your mind occupied with those books or movies that you have on hand and planning that wonderful new life free from drugs that you have in front of you.

Believe you can and you're halfway there. -Theodore Roosevelt

After Detox - Stop the Madness Merry-Go-Round

I don't need help quitting, I have quite a thousand times! I need help STAYING QUIT! - The White Book

If this is your first go around with a Detox experience, be glad that it's over. Don't stop reading though as there are some important things that you need to consider, some "hard facts" if you will. If you've been through this before, the following will likely not come as much of a surprise to you, yet the reminders may do you some good and, hopefully, send you in the right direction this time. The fact of the matter is that simply getting the drugs and/or alcohol out of our system isn't enough to recover from addiction.

Many of us, myself included, have suffered from the delusions that we were simply trapped in a "physical addiction" and, once free, would be able to resume living life just as we had before all of this nonsense started. Wrong! There is an "invisible line" that has been crossed and you will never be able to go back to that "old life". That's the bad news. The good news is that you absolutely can recover from this and lead an even better life than you had ever imagined. Yes, it sounds ridiculous and like a bunch of "hocus pocus" right now, but stick with me here. There is light at the end of the tunnel after a bit more education and self discovery.

Who is Molly

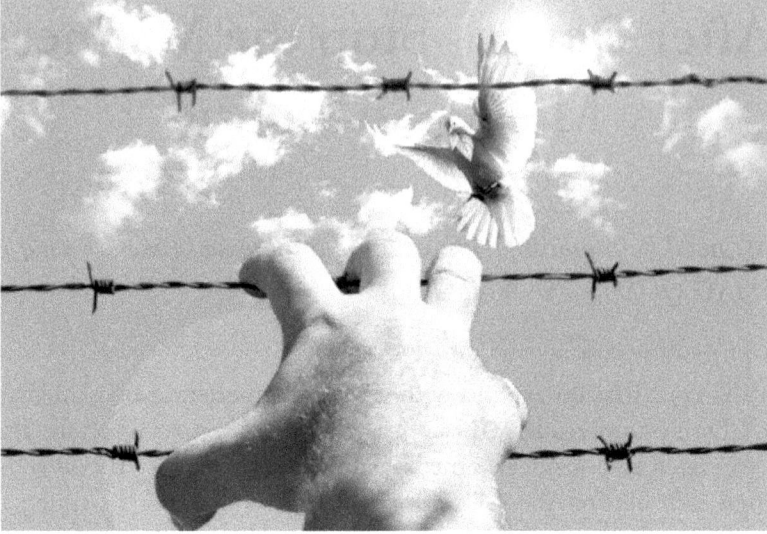

Addiction As a Disease

Whether you sniff it smoke it eat it or shove it up your ass the result is the same: addiction. -William S. Burroughs

A fact that most addicts and alcoholics are in the dark about is that they actually have a "disease" and are not simply bad people that can't control themselves. In fact, for over 100 years, alcoholism has been treated as and defined as a "disease". In 1956, the American Medical Association voted to define alcoholism as a disease and, according to the National Institute on Drug Abuse (NIDA), "Addiction is defined as a chronic, relapsing brain disease that is characterized by compulsive drug seeking and use, despite harmful consequences." The American Society of Addiction Medicine (ASAM) also recently revised its definition of addiction to state that: "Addiction is a chronic brain disorder, and not merely a behavioral problem or simply the result of taking the wrong choices". Addiction is now described as a primary disease - not caused by something else, such as a psychiatric or emotional problem.   Dr. Michael Miller, former president of ASAM, who oversaw the development of the new definition, said: "At its core, addiction isn't just a social problem or a moral problem or a criminal problem. It's a brain problem whose behaviors manifest in all these other areas. Many behaviors driven by addiction are real problems and sometimes criminal acts. But the disease is about brains, not drugs. It's about underlying neurology, not outward actions."

Who is Molly

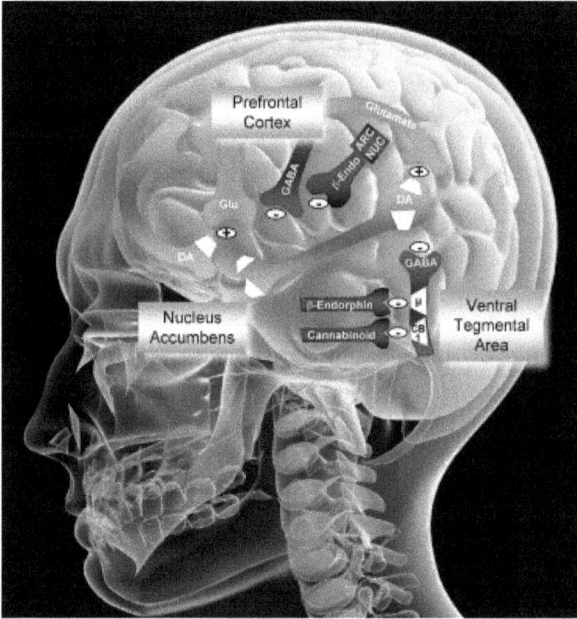

A few additional characteristics of the disease of Addiction (and Alcoholism - same thing) to be aware of are:

Mental Obsession - Defined as a thought process over which you have no control. Sounds like fun, right? These maddening urges to use or drink, when many times we know that the results will be disastrous. I always call this the "preoccupation" that I always had with when I would be able to get that next drink or drug - or how I would be able to get more than my "share".

Chronic Disease - By chronic, we mean that it is "incurable" (keep reading anyway) and requires long-term treatment. This is a disease that can also result in death if not treated.

Progressive - This one is important. Well, the other two were also. Addiction and Alcoholism is a subtly progressive disease that gets worse over time - NEVER better. Sometimes, this takes place over such an extended period of time that the addict does not notice the point at which they truly lost control. And, you know what? It doesn't matter. Because as soon as that control is "lost", it can NEVER be regained. EVER. This is where the difficulty and the denial come into play for so many. We remember that time when things were great, fun, easy, controllable and try with all our might, sometimes for entirely too long, to recapture it. It just won't happen.

So what does all of this new-found knowledge mean for the "addicted" or stricken person? Well, the good news is that you're "sick"! Yes, in this case, consider this good news. Think of it in these terms: you no longer need look at yourself as a bad person or an evil person who has screwed up their life and can't control themselves. The truth is that you are a "sick person" who simply needs to take some steps to get well. This is entirely possible and well within your reach if it is something that you want. While there is no cure per se for addiction, this is a disease that you can recover from and lead a happy, healthy and productive life. However, if you think that you had to do a little bit of self seeking and self discovery before jumping into a detox situation, that was a cake walk. Reaching a point of "surrender" and starting the road to recovery requires that you be willing to honestly take a look at yourself and take some action.

End-stage addiction is mostly about waiting for the police, or someone, to come and bury you in your shame. — David Carr

Who is Molly

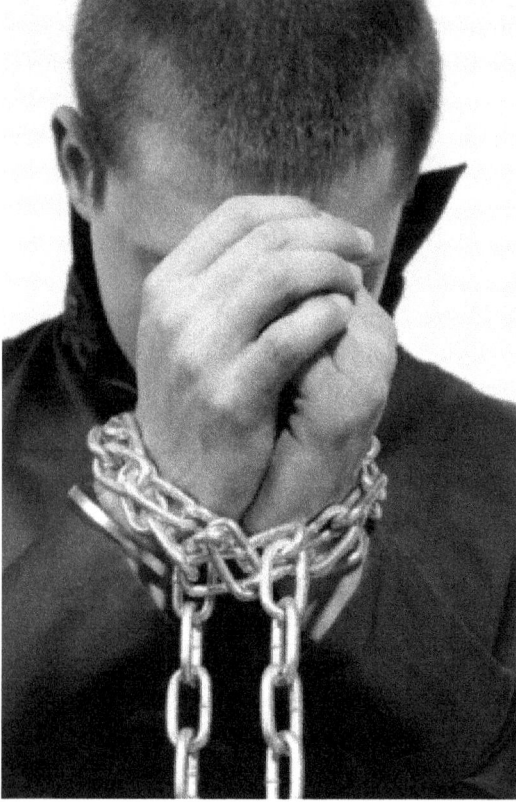

Hitting a Bottom with Molly

When you're drowning, you don't say 'I would be incredibly pleased if someone would have the foresight to notice me drowning and come and help me,' you just scream. -John Lennon

Hopefully you asked yourself this question before you put yourself through any sort of detox. What's important to understand here is that for most of us, drugs and alcohol provided some sort of benefits in the beginning and for potentially a long period of time in our lives. Then, at some point, negative consequences of using and drinking started to accumulate and, either it just wasn't fun anymore, it wasn't working anymore, or the consequences were too painful to want to continue using. Regardless, many of us call this a "bottom" and you should take some time to try to define what your bottom is and how it could (and would) get worse should you continue to use.

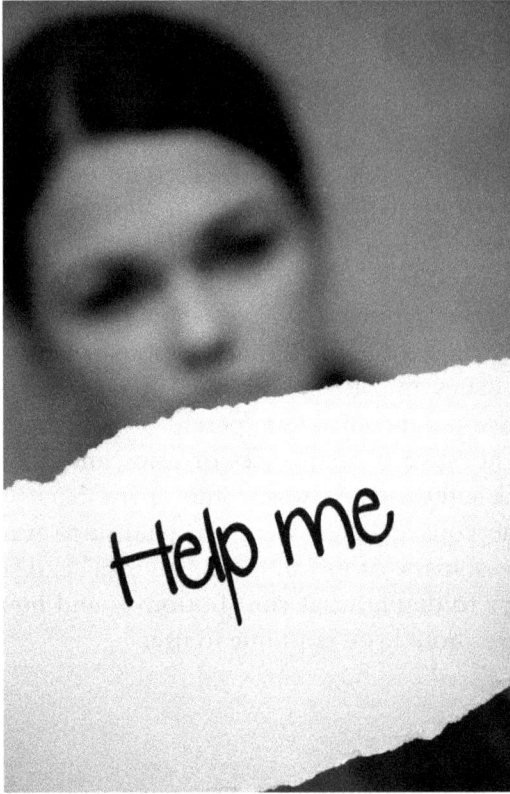

Unfortunately, addicts and alcoholics are characterized by extreme arrogance and stubbornness. This is why many of us have multiple "bottoms" - where we stop using and think that we can control our drinking and using so decide to give it another try. I can tell you from experience and from observing countless others that things always get worse and that attempts to control an addiction are, in the end, futile. Sometimes deadly. The fact of the matter is this - we can chose our bottom. This can be it - right now.

Should I Go to Treatment?

...we do not always like what is good for us in this world. -Eleanor Roosevelt

Most addicts and alcoholics assume that they have to go to treatment to get better. I did and ended up in an endless stream of rehabs. In fact, if you spend any time in front of the television (most do), then we are taught that in order to "get sober", you have to go to rehab. This isn't necessarily the case and the treatment center industry has seen a recent "boom" in the past few decades as getting sober is now all the rage. So, are these fancy places necessary to start your road to recovery? This is hotly debated and the answer is different for each individual. Many people are able to get clean and sober and stay that way with the help of 12 Step programs alone - no rehab. However, in our fast paced society with all of life's demands, treatment centers certainly have carved out their niche in the "getting sober" process and have some very real value.

It may be that you haven't been given a choice. The edict to "go to rehab" could have been handed down by an employer, a family member or even a judge. If that's the case, the question has been answered for you. Otherwise, if you are still pondering whether or not to go to treatment, there are several different types of treatment centers to choose from and they certainly do have their benefits if you decide to go.

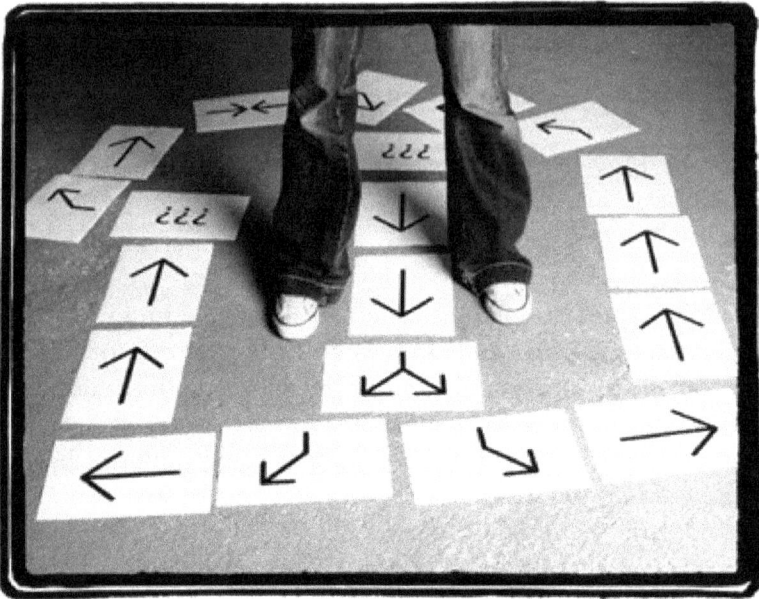

At fifteen life had taught me undeniably that surrender, in its place, was as honorable as resistance, especially if one had no choice. - *Maya Angelou*

Different Types of Treatment Centers

I have found that sitting in a place where you have never sat before can be inspiring. -Dodie Smith

Choices abound as to what sort of treatment center, if any, is going to be right for you. You will need to decide between Inpatient or Outpatient, Private or Public and, in some cases, Co-Ed or Single Sex treatment centers.

Inpatient vs Outpatient - Many people are inclined to select "outpatient" right off the bat because we are also inclined to downplay the seriousness of our situation and the means necessary to recover from it. Some people are able to successfully participate in treatment programs on a part-time basis while continuing to live at home, manage their family lives and keep their jobs. These people are exceptions to the rule, however. There are other outpatient treatment programs that simply have you go to treatment during the day and return to your home (and family) at night. Again, depending on your circumstances, this may be a viable option. For many, and for a lot of reasons, it's not for a lot of people.

Inpatient drug and alcohol treatment is more the norm for quite a few reasons. This option dictates that the individual moves into some sort of dorm-like setting and receives 24/7 care and supervision. Some treatment centers allow for private and semi-private rooms, while others you will essentially take what you are given. Inpatient treatment is the ideal choice for someone who needs a place to focus entirely on their addiction and developing their recovery program.

Private vs Public - Regardless of the previous differences, you will run into rehab centers that are both Private and Publicly funded. Different treatment funding sources include:

- Private: Non-profit, or For Profit
- State or Locally Funded

- Low Cost Treatment Centers
- Free Rehabs (Charity Rehabs)

While the Free, Low Cost and Government Funded treatment centers sound great (they are, I got sober in one), it's important to note that many also have long waiting lists. Another difference, although not true in all cases, may be the size of groups in therapy sessions, with smaller groups in Private facilities and larger groups in publicly funded rehabs. Also, do not expect to get into any sort of private or semi-private room in a public facility. In retrospect, being "pampered" did nothing to get me sober. I did find the many waiting lists very disheartening though when I was finally "ready" for this and just couldn't get in anyplace. So, if you are looking at Private treatment centers and possible ways to finance it, consider these:

- **Health Insurance** - most "good" health insurance policies provide for some form of substance abuse treatment. If you have a really good policy, you may be able to get an inpatient treatment program paid for
- **Family Members** - you may already have family members offering to pay to get you sober. I did. I even had friends of family willing to chip in at one point.
- **Sell stock or take money from your 401k** - If you're unemployed, in jail or dead, there will be no "retirement" to save for, right?
- **Home Equity Loan** - If you are lucky enough to still be holding onto your home, consider this.
- **Sell stuff, even your car** - Chances are you have expensive toys you haven't been using because of you've been putting all of your efforts into drugging and partying. Sell them. You don't need a car if you're not sober. It's a hazard.
- **Substance Abuse Treatment Loan** - Yes, they have these now.

Co-ed vs Same Sex Treatment Centers - I've been to both and it didn't make a difference to me either way. However, if you have been the victim of abuse and think that you would feel safer in a same sex facility, by all means, check them out.

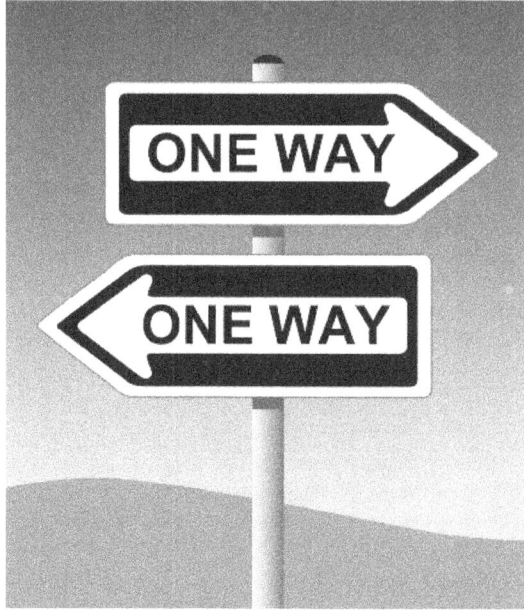

It's not how far you fall, but how high you bounce that counts. -Zig Ziglar

The Pros and Cons of Going to Rehab

A man's errors are his portals of discovery. -James Joyce

When I first started hitting the treatment centers, I didn't see any "Pro's" to this nonsense whatsoever. I did not want to be there, did not think that I had a problem like the rest of the folks in that place did and felt very inconvenienced by the whole thing. Quite a few treatment centers and many years of sobriety later, it's much easier to see their benefit. However, I do clearly see what the Con's are in committing to these institutions. Here are a few:

Con's of Going to Treatment

Time - Yes, you are committing a substantial amount of your time to this program. You are committing literally ALL of your time if you elect to go to an inpatient treatment center. This means that family and work responsibilities need to be re-arranged. In many cases, some or all of those have "dissolved" on their own because of our drinking and drugging activities.

Cost - Most people would agree that this is the biggest downside to treatment, particularly private rehabs. Inpatient programs can cost upwards of $1,000 per day and outpatient programs are not cheap either. Publicly funded programs are more affordable but there are oftentimes many hoops to jump through to qualify and get into these programs.

Pro's of Going to Treatment

Structured Environment - One of the biggest benefits of attending treatment, primarily residential (or inpatient), is that you are provided with a safe, structured environment that is free of distractions and temptations. This will give you a window of opportunity to get clean and sober (post-detox) and learn how to live life without drugs and alcohol. This structured environment is designed to essentially be free of the daily stressors of work, home and family so that you can focus only on your recovery.

Establish Network of Positive People - Attending treatment, inpatient or outpatient, gives you the opportunity to form new friendships and bonds with other like-minded, positive people. These are relationships that can be the beginning of your sober support network.

Learning Better Holistic Health - If giving up drinking and drugs were enough, this would be a much shorter book. However, the real purpose of recovery is to learn how to live a happy and healthy life without drugs and alcohol. Learning to treat yourself well in all respects in something that you can learn in treatment, such as eating right, being physically active and taking care of your mental and spiritual well-being.

Save Money - Wait, what?! Didn't we just say in the "Con's" that "cost" was a downside to going to treatment? Well, yes we did. BUT, let's look at the big picture here. The amount of money that you will save in long run by getting, and staying sober, is astounding compared to continuing with that financial minefield of active addiction. Many people are blown away when they see the financial figures tied to their disease. I'm not just talking about the money spent on drugs and alcohol (count this, though). Add in jobs lost, promotions lost, missed opportunities, legal fees, smashed cars, foreclosed homes, and so on. Looking at it this way, the cost of a stint at that fancy rehab may not look as outrageous as it did earlier.

Save Your Life - For some, it really does boil down to this. It's simply a matter of life or death. Without some real, structured help, the end is imminent. A lot of addicts and alcoholics run to treatment in hopes that they will "save" something or get their lives back. What many find is that they have been given an entirely new life that is infinitely better than anything they could have ever dreamed possible.

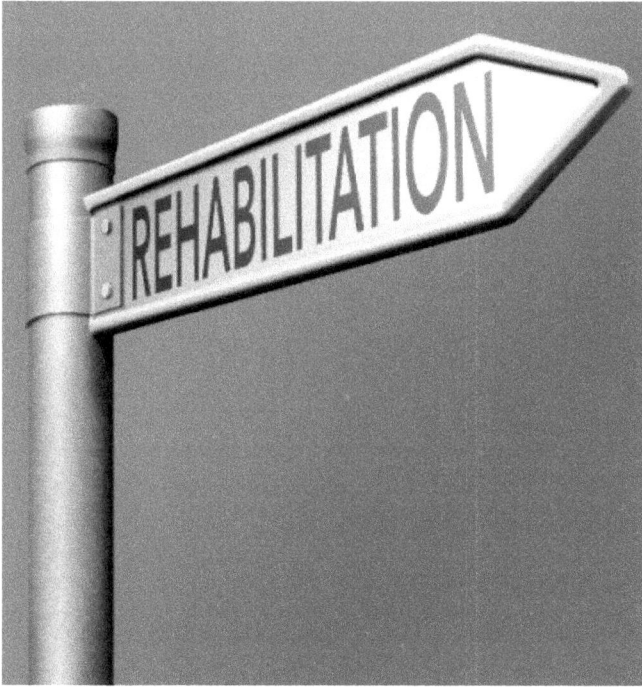

The best way out is always through. —Robert Frost

Making the Most of Rehab If You Decide to Go

Asking for help does not mean that we are weak or incompetent. It usually indicates an advanced level of honesty and intelligence. -Jim Rohn

If you make the decision to go to a treatment facility, good for you! You are giving yourself a gift that will not only come back to you tenfold but to those you know and love as well, even if your relationships aren't as you would want them to be right now. As we reviewed earlier, there are so many different types of treatment facilities so it's not possible to give you a perfect run down of what to expect. However, here are a few words of wisdom so that you can make the most of your stay:

There will be no locks on the doors. This doesn't work, not even for a second, if you're not willing so you can walk away at any time. Even if you are court ordered to be at a place, they'll just come and pick you up to face your consequences at a later date should you bolt. Check your willingness level at the door, and thereafter frequently, and commit to stay for whatever term is recommended.

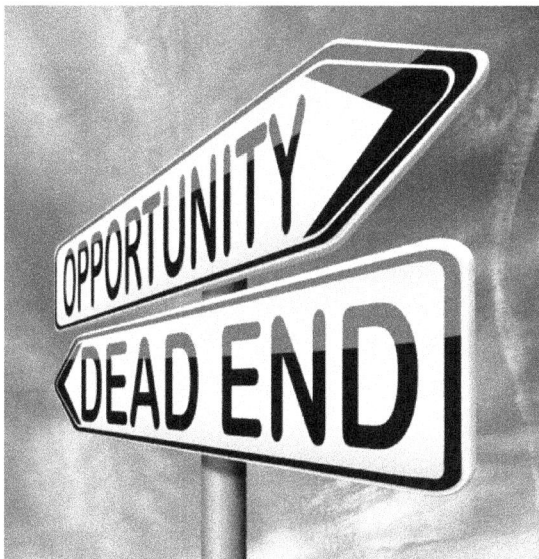

Who is Molly

If you go - From my experience with the revolving doors of many treatment centers, these are my words of wisdom. First and foremost, check the attitude at the door. This is one thing that I took in with me and held onto through nearly all of my stays, except for the last one. It did me no favors. Thinking that I still knew what was best for me, after the shit storm that I had just made of my life was ludicrous. Also, demanding that I be given respect and attention when I felt I needed it was just as insane. I had to come to a place where I finally understood that I knew absolutely nothing about how to recover from this disease and that these people were clearly authorities on the subject. So probably, I should just let them do their job and listen to someone else for a change. Once I did this - made this mental shift (some would call it "surrender"), going to treatment was a blessing for me and I made the most of every single opportunity that was put in front of me to learn and to start my recovery. Yes, this included going to AA, which I also resisted for a long time.

When we are no longer able to change a situation - we are challenged to change ourselves. Viktor E. Frankl

Support Groups

Separate reeds are easily broken; but bound together they are strong and hard to break apart. -The Midrash

Yes, we are talking about a 12 Step Group here, NA or AA preferably. There are alternative "recovery groups" out there but this author knows absolutely nothing about them or their success rates. What I do know is that 12 Step Groups work 100% for people that follow the directions 100%. That's the key. Many people, myself included, have avoided getting sober simply because they feared "joining" AA or NA. I had no concept of what this group was or just how something like this could possibly be of any assistance to me. I didn't understand what AA was and there is always the fear of the unknown. I speak mostly about AA because that is what I attend. Despite my long history of drug use and abuse, I have found that AA takes care of everything for me and so have many others.

So, what is AA then? What it is, really, is a multi-faceted program that incorporates meetings, fellowship and working a 12-step program in order to bring about a change in the alcoholic and provide continued growth and support. (NA is the same - they just change some words around in the "steps" and the literature is different.) AA was founded in 1935 by Bill Wilson (known as Bill W) and Dr. Robert Smith (known as Dr. Bob), based on the main principle of one alcoholic sharing their experiences with another. Within 4 years, their basic text called "Alcoholics Anonymous" (aka The Big Book) was published and membership blossomed. Today, there are over 2 million members of AA world-wide (over 1/2 of these in the U.S.) and over 115,000 registered AA Groups. In fact, there are now over 200 different fellowships that employ the "12 Steps" for recovery from AA (altered to fit). Hard to argue with those numbers.

Giving up control is difficult and joining a "Support Group" of any sort is giving up another layer of control with respect to this disease. Believe me - I get it. I had to get to a place in my life and with my disease where I finally understood that my way wasn't working in any way, shape or form and I became willing to try something else. Recovery from addiction happens on many levels: physical, mental, emotional and spiritual. The program of AA addresses these different levels of recovery through it's different facets of: attending meetings, getting a sponsor, working the 12 steps, spiritual principles and involvement in the fellowship. In doing these things, old habits are broken, new (healthy) habits are formed, and we are able to take a deeper look at the causes and conditions underlying our long drinking and using careers. All of this is done in some manner that taps into the mechanisms that counter the complex neurological and psychological processes through which this disease wreaks its havoc. Better yet, it's done through the power of "the group". Psychologists have long known that one of the best ways to change human behavior is to gather people with similar problems into groups instead of treating them individually. This is one of AA's precepts.

Whether it is the initial act of "surrender", the group support setting, the self-awareness that comes from working the Steps, or the close relationships in the fellowship through helping others that are the key components to the alcoholic's recovery (one or all of these), no one knows. What we do know, however, is that despite all we've learned over the past few decades about psychology, neurology, and human behavior, contemporary medicine has yet to devise anything that works markedly better. "In my 20 years of treating addicts, I've never seen anything else that comes close to the 12 steps," says Drew Pinsky, the addiction-medicine specialist who hosts VH1's Celebrity Rehab. While AA may not be a miracle cure for all, people who become deeply involved in the program stay clean and sober and do well over the long haul, and this starts with attending meetings. Check out the Resources Section at the end of the book for links to various 12 Step Groups. It starts by attendance at the first meeting and goes from there. Addiction is not something that can, or should, be battled alone.

There are no problems we cannot solve together, and very few that we can solve by ourselves. -Lyndon B. Johnson

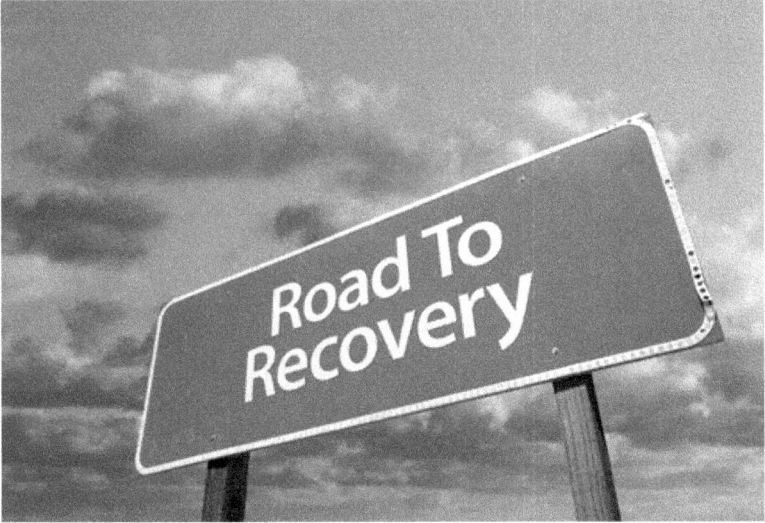

Talking to Your Teen or Loved One About Molly

There is no such thing as a problem without a gift for you in its hands. -Richard Bach

As parents, it's often tough to approach certain sensitive subjects with our children. When is the right time? How young is too young? How should I discuss it? But given the rise in popularity of Molly, the time to talk to your teen about the drug and its dangers is now. Experts recommend talking to your kids about drugs early and often. No kidding, the conversation starts at age two. By the time your children are 16 to 18, says the website DrugFree.org, they will likely already have had to make choices about drug use. They will likely already have seen peers using alcohol and drugs.

"They all know about it. They're talking about it, and a fair amount of young people are experimenting with it," explains Jeffrey Reynolds, Ph.D., Executive Director of the Long Island Council on Alcoholism and Drug Dependence. When talking to your teen about Molly, Reynolds encourages parents to keep the conversation light, starting by asking them if they've ever heard about the drug or know of anyone who's tried it, gauging their general knowledge of the substance. Stress the dangers of drug use as well as the potential hazards related to Molly, specifically, being sure to include drinking in the conversation, as most encounters with the drug usually begin with alcohol. Even if your teen isn't using the drug, chances are they know someone who is, so arming them with the information they need can still save a life. After all, one of the most powerful forms of prevention against drug and alcohol use is knowledge.

Who is Molly

It is very likely that, if your child is pre-teen or older, they may have already heard of Molly, although the younger tweens may not be entirely clear on what it is. The Miley Cyrus song "We Can't Stop" is a great place to start as it includes lyrics about "dancing with Molly" and is, in fact, about "rolling" and using MDMA. Talk about the song with your teen and perhaps discuss the fact that Ms. Cyrus is no longer the positive role model that she used to be, pointing out the fact that she can't even seem to keep her tongue inside her mouth and her clothes on anymore.

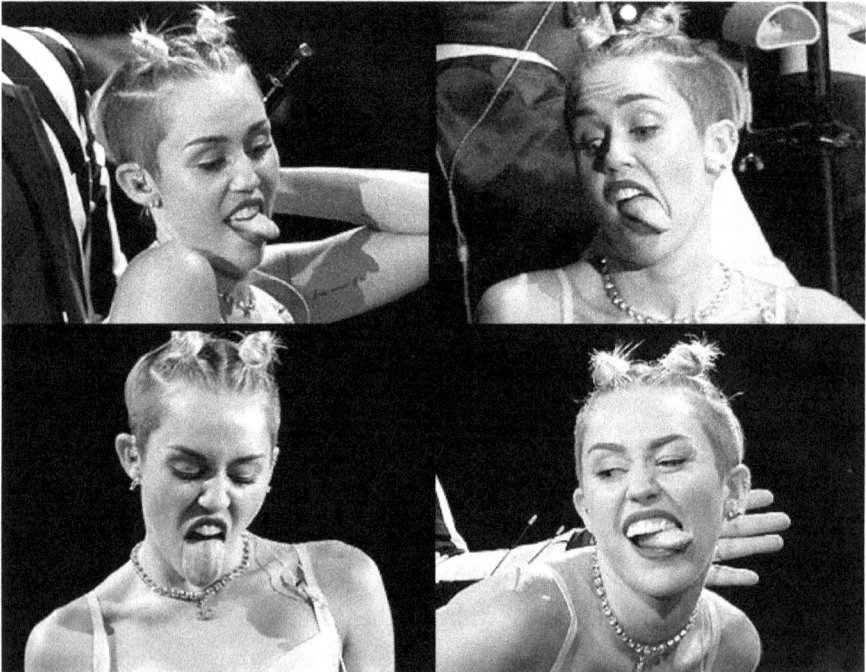

Showing pictures of the drugs to your kids is a good idea, too. Ecstasy, for example, is oftentimes pressed into pills and made to look like candy. The more specific you can be with your kids, the better. Talk about what's been shared in the news and give details. It's a good idea to explain why this stuff can be dangerous and make it easy for them to relate to. Sure, MDMA reportedly makes people feel good (for a while), but it's impossible to know how an individual's brain is going to react to the drug – and to the come-down. If there are any medical conditions in the family, explain how these can be dangerous when combined with a street drug. In addition, if there is a history of drug and alcohol addiction in the family, stress this each time you talk about drugs with your child.

I have a 15 year-old son and we talk about drugs and alcohol often. We always have. Some of the things that we talk about are peer pressure, the current drug trends in his schools and my personal experiences with drugs and alcohol. Being in recovery, I have long history of making bad decisions and I can share with my son the stories of the years of pain and loss that those decisions created. All decisions – good and bad – have repercussions. I know that my child will make bad decisions sometimes, because everyone makes bad decisions sometimes. It's part of being human, and it's definitely part of growing up. Sometimes bad decisions end up hurting someone's feelings, for example. Sometimes we might choose not to study very much, and then we don't do well on a test. I was lucky and was able to turn my life around before it was too late. The thing is to try not to make the bad decisions that can make you dead.

So, how do you know if your teen is using Molly? Well, if you have recently heard your teen talking with his or her friends about their new friend Molly, then you might want to stick your nose into their business – at least a little. If your child walks through your door and something seems "off," look for these signs:

* Jaw clenching

- No appetite
- High and low temperatures
- Mood swings
- Large pupils
- Confusion
- Sleep problems
- Profuse sweating
- Rapid eye movement
- Memory loss
- Blurred vision

Take these with a grain of salt and look at the entire picture, however. My teen exhibits several of these signs on a daily basis and I know he's not using Molly. However, if your teen is exhibiting a number of these signs together and you are unsure, it's important to seek medical help. Have them checked out at the emergency room to ensure their health and safety. These are short-term reactions, so it's important to look at the total picture. If your teen has been skipping school, changing friends, experiencing mood swings or lacking proper sleep and eating habits, these could be signs of a drug addiction.

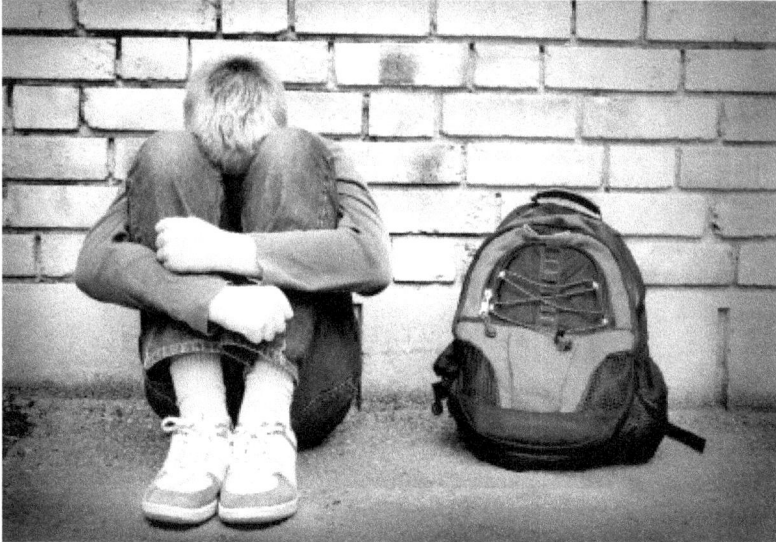

Parents need to be proactive. It's not just noticing the signs of Molly use, but also teaching your child the dangers of taking the drug. Because frankly, if you just tell your kids "don't do drugs," that's not really very helpful. If parents don't speak up, kids start learning about the world from music and movies, and we know where that leads. Unfortunately, many parents are unaware of Molly, so it's difficult to warn your kids about something you don't know exists. Look for additional sources of help in talking to your children and teen about drugs and alcohol in the Useful Resources section at the end of the book.

It is astonishing in this world how things don't turn out at all the way you expect them to! -Agatha Christie

Useful Resources

There are no "public" websites that offer treatment center, detox and sober living directories. Unfortunately, any site you find will be filled with "sponsored results". This means rehabs that have paid for ad space. That's not always a bad thing, just not an unbiased thing. The best site I've found is Sober.com. You'll get the sponsored results in your search but you will also get all of the public listings as well, including the government-funded (some free) facilities.

Another Treatment Center Resource (drugrehabcenters.org)
This one also lists the treatment centers that either have a sliding fee scale, accept public funds or are free.

Support Groups

Alcoholics Anonymous (aa.org)
Al-Anon Websites (al-anon.alateen.org)
Narcotics Anonymous (na.org)
Cocaine Anonymous (ca.org)
Adult Children of Alcoholics (adultchildren.org)
Co-Dependence Anonymous (CoDA) (coda.org)

Ecstasy Resources

Dance Safe (dancesafe.org)
Safety Information and MDMA Test Kits

Ecstasydata.org
EcstasyData.org is an independent laboratory pill testing program co-sponsored by Erowid, Dancesafe, and Isomer Deseign. Launched in July 2001, its purpose is to collect, manage, review, and present laboratory pill testing results from a variety of organizations.

Pill Reports (pillreports.com)
Pillreports is a global database of "Ecstasy" pills based on both subjective user reports and scientific analysis. By identifying dangerous adulterants, Pillreports performs a vital harm reduction service that can prevent many of the problems associated with "Ecstasy" use before they happen.

NEWIP (Nightlife Empowerment & Well-being Implementation Project) (safernightlife.org)
NEWIP is carried out by a network of European community-based NGOs acting in the nightlife field, nightlife professionals, local and regional authorities and agencies, treatment professionals and scientific researchers. The NEWIP partnership is based on the alliance of the Basics Network with the Democracy, Cities & Drugs Safer Nightlife Platform: Created in 1998, the members of the Basics Network "for dance culture and drug awareness" are European peer projects issued from party scenes with the aim of promoting health and harm reduction in the recreational settings.

Other Ecstasy Test Kits

Bunk Police Test Kit (bunkpolice.org/basic-test-kit/)

EZ Test Ecstasy Test Kit (eztest.com)

Home Drug Testing Kits for MDMA (test your teen)

Test Country Single MDMA Test (testcountry.com)

TeenSavers Multi-Drug Test

Mental Health

National Institute of Mental Health (nimh.nih.gov)
Results of biomedical research on mind and behavior.

National Alliance for the Mentally Ill (nami.org)
Support for consumers with mental illness

Substance Abuse & Mental Health Services Administration (samhsa.gov)
United States Department of Health & Human Services

Multidisciplinary Association for Psychedelic Studies (MAPS) (maps.org)
Founded in 1986, the Multidisciplinary Association for Psychedelic Studies (MAPS) is a 501(c)(3) non-profit research and educational organization that develops medical, legal, and cultural contexts for people to benefit from the careful uses of psychedelics and marijuana. MAPS is currently studying whether MDMA-assisted psychotherapy has the potential to heal the psychological and emotional damage

caused by sexual assault, war, violent crime, and other traumas.

Government Resources

Single-State Agency (SSA) Directory: Prevention and Treatment of Substance Use and Mental Disorders – A list of State offices that can provide local information and guidance about substance use and mental disorders, treatment, and recovery in your community.

AMVETS (amvets.org)
This organization provides support for veterans and the active military in procuring their earned entitlements. It also offers community services that enhance the quality of life for this Nation's citizens.

Professionals

Intervention Project for Nurses (ipnfl.org)
Help   for   professionals   with   chemical   dependencies.

International Lawyers in Alcoholics Anonymous (ILAA) (ilaa.org)
This organization serves as a clearinghouse for support groups for lawyers who are recovering from alcohol or other chemical dependencies.

International   Pharmacists   Anonymous   (IPA)
(home.comcast.net/~mitchfields/ipa/ipapage.htm)
This is a 12-step fellowship of pharmacists and pharmacy students recovering   from   any   addiction.

Other

The Parent Toolkit (theparenttoolkit.org)
A drug and alcohol prevention resource for parents.

NIDA for Teens (teens.drugabuse.gov)
The National Institute on Drug Abuse (NIDA), a component of the National Institutes of Health (NIH), created this Web site to educate adolescents ages 11 through 15 (as well as their parents and teachers) on the science behind drug abuse. NIDA enlisted the help of teens in developing the site to ensure that the content addresses appropriate questions and timely concerns.

AlcoholScreening.org - Website offering an online screening tool to assess drinking patterns. The website offers visitors free confidential online screenings to assess their drinking patterns, giving them personalized feedback and showing them if their alcohol consumption is likely to be within safe limits. AlcoholScreening.org was developed by Join Together, a project of the Boston University School of Public Health, and was launched in April 2001. The website also provides answers to frequently asked questions about alcohol and health consequences, and provides links to support resources and a database of local treatment programs. Disclaimer: This site does not provide a diagnosis of alcohol abuse, alcohol dependence or any other medical condition. The information provided here cannot substitute for a full evaluation by a health professional, and should only be used as a guide to understanding your alcohol use and the potential health issues involved with it.

This Center for Substance Abuse Prevention widget includes a variety of updates on activities relating to underage drinking which is updated regularly with local, state, and national articles published by online sources.

NCADD (ncadd.org):

The National Council on Alcoholism and Drug Dependence, Inc. (NCADD) and its Affiliate Network is a voluntary health organization dedicated to fighting the Nation's #1 health problem – alcoholism, drug addiction and the devastating consequences of alcohol and other drugs on individuals, families and communities.

American Council for Drug Education (acde.org)

Educational programs and services for teens, parents, and educators

About the Author

Taite Adams is a successful marketer and published author who has traded in the high cost of low living for a much more peaceful, and rewarding, life. Free of alcohol and drugs for over a decade and an active member of Alcoholics Anonymous, Taite (not her real name) enjoys living a sober life and sharing those joys with her family, friends and people looking for a better way to live. She is an avid boater, licensed Coast Guard Captain and prolific traveler. While her bucket list remains long, each day brings a shining new opportunity to cross something off the list or discover something new - and for that she remains forever grateful.

As you gather valuable information on addiction or begin your Road to Recovery, please check out Taite's other book, Kickstart Your Recovery, available in both Kindle and Paperback.

Should you require additional assistance with your home detox, be sure to pick up Taite's popular book, Safely Detox From Alcohol and Drugs at Home, also on Amazon.com.

Opiate Addiction has reached epidemic proportions in this country and is something that Taite is intimately familiar with. Read her latest book, that is climbing the charts on Amazon, chronicling this insidious killer and laying the pathway for freedom from its grip.

If you or a loved one are in recovery from alcoholism or addiction and want to learn more about emotional sobriety, check out Taite's latest book titled Restart Your Recovery, also on Amazon.com.

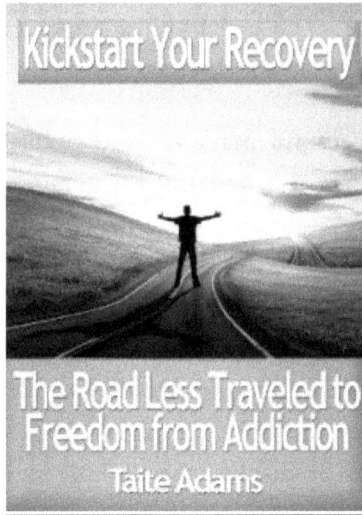

Kickstart Your Recovery
The Road Less Traveled to Freedom from Addiction
Taite Adams

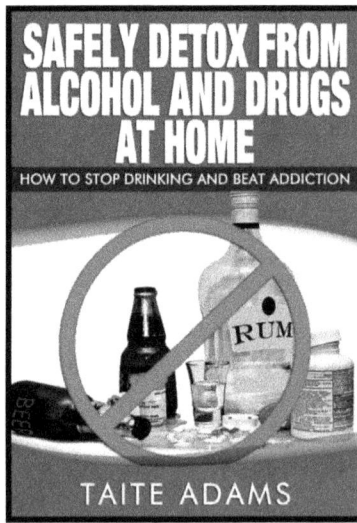

SAFELY DETOX FROM ALCOHOL AND DRUGS AT HOME
HOW TO STOP DRINKING AND BEAT ADDICTION
TAITE ADAMS

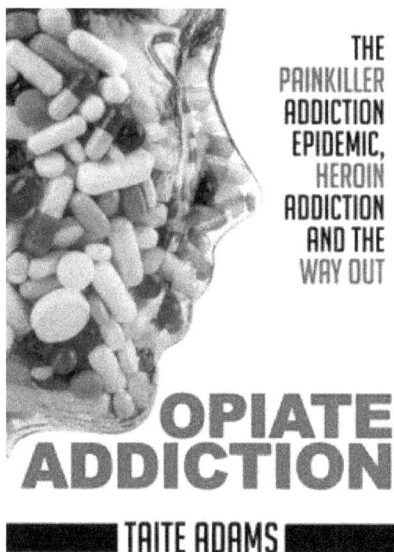

THE
PAINKILLER
ADDICTION
EPIDEMIC,
HEROIN
ADDICTION
AND THE
WAY OUT

OPIATE
ADDICTION

TAITE ADAMS

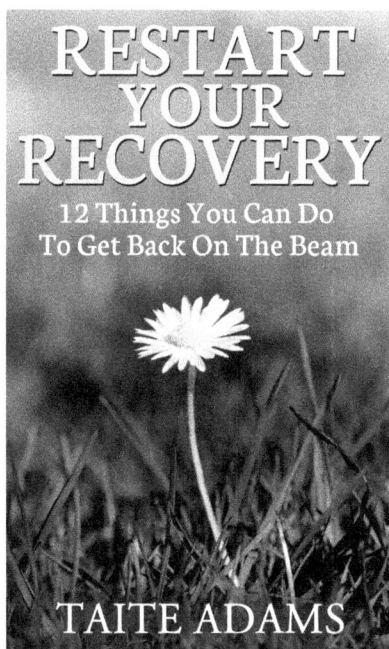

RESTART
YOUR
RECOVERY

12 Things You Can Do
To Get Back On The Beam

TAITE ADAMS

For More Information, Visit
http://www.taiteadams.com

www.ingramcontent.com/pod-product-compliance
Lightning Source LLC
Chambersburg PA
CBHW061750020426
42331CB00006B/1415